FUTURECARE

REFLEX ARC

FUTURECARE
New Directions in Planning Health and Care Environments

edited by

MARTIN S. VALINS
BA(Hons), DipArch., RIBA

and

DEREK SALTER
DipArch.(Oxford), RIBA

**Blackwell
Science**

© 1996 by
Blackwell Science Ltd
Editorial Offices:
Osney Mead, Oxford OX2 0EL
25 John Street, London WC1N 2BL
23 Ainslie Place, Edinburgh EH3 6AJ
238 Main Street, Cambridge
  Massachusetts 02142, USA
54 University Street, Carlton
  Victoria 3053, Australia

Other Editorial Offices:
Arnette Blackwell SA
  224, Boulevard Saint Germain
  75007 Paris, France

Blackwell Wissenschafts-Verlag GmbH
  Kurfürstendamm 57
  10707 Berlin, Germany

  Zehetnergasse 6
  A-1140 Wien
  Austria

First published 1996

Set in 10 on 12½ pt Century Book
by DP Photosetting, Aylesbury, Bucks

DISTRIBUTORS

Marston Book Services Ltd
PO Box 269
Abingdon
Oxford OX14 4YN
(*Orders*: Tel: 01235 46550
         Fax: 01235 46555)

USA
Blackwell Science, Inc.
238 Main Street
Cambridge, MA 02142
(*Orders*: Tel: 800 215-1000
         617 876-7000
         Fax: 617 492-5263)

Canada
Copp Clark, Ltd
2775 Matheson Blvd East
Mississauga, Ontario
Canada, L4W 4P7
(*Orders*: Tel: 800 263-4374
         905 238-6074)

Australia
Blackwell Science Pty Ltd
54 University Street
Carlton, Victoria 3053
(*Orders*: Tel: 03 9347 0300
         Fax: 03 9349 3016)

A catalogue record for this title
is available from the British Library

ISBN 0–632–03577–3

Library of Congress
Cataloging-in-Publication Data
is available

Contents

We shape our buildings: thereafter they shape us.

Sir Winston Churchill
(*Time*, September 12, 1960)

Preface

In the preparation of this book, we aimed to involve and invite as wide a spectrum of opinion as possible to envisage what a future healthcare landscape might consist of. We do not propose a single path to the future but instead an ordered variety of informed comment and opinion. The debate as to how healthcare is financed and developed has been, and always will be, an ongoing challenge. Our task therefore has been to identify those core issues which are driving change.

This book is simply laid out as a series of themes which we consider important to the future care debate. Each theme is interconnected with the others. Some issues which are discussed may well reappear elsewhere in the book. Some contradict. This is deliberate. Reading through the book one will discover common threads of argument – the underlying trends of future care that form the fabric of the key issues that we all need to be aware of in planning for the future.

This book is about change, and the revolution that is currently taking place in the various ways in which health care is delivered to our communities.

It is not about how to design buildings for health and care. There are already many excellent publications available. Instead this book focuses upon what providers of health and care environments should be considering in order to be aware of current trends and to anticipate those in the future. As such *Futurecare* is not so much a practical desktop manual, it is a book which steps back to offer an overview: not to contemplate the footprints on the sand but to be prepared for the coming tidal wave.

Futurecare will therefore describe new directions that will shape future generations of buildings designed to accommodate health and care programmes into the next century. It aims to provide an insight for all those concerned in the development, design, administration and management of health and care buildings. Its focus will be to define what must be considered today in order to prepare for the radically changing needs of tomorrow.

Futurecare is not concerned with crystal ball gazing. Events do not happen in a vacuum but in social, political, cultural and economic contexts. Future trends do not appear overnight. They are often the result of decades or more of subtle influences and events which eventually shape future policy and direction. Like a tidal wave, the impact of future change can appear instantly dramatic yet its causes can often be traced back to past events, often years in the making. This book therefore describes and examines the origins of current health and care facility planning in order to detect those influences which will shape the future.

For hundreds of years the year 2000 has stood for the future. In a few short years that future will have arrived. The impending dawn of this new millennium will focus attention on what lies beyond the Rubicon between old and new, present and future. The consequences of past policies and often myopic approaches to planning health and care facilities have become apparent, particularly in recent times. As a result the debate as to the type of services and facilities which will be required in the future has intensified.

The subject of that debate throughout the developed world is how future care planning can be in tune with and sensitive to future needs of the market. Health and care planners should ensure that what they plan for today will not be redundant in the near future. Conference agendas and professional journals all talk of 'tomorrow'. Perhaps the process of planning health and care environments has more long-term implications than any other activity. Any building developed for healthcare will typically be utilized for its intended purpose for many decades.

Any new building therefore by implication may need to provide future care far beyond the original planning horizons. Anyone involved in the process of planning for health and care carries a responsibility for playing a part in determining future care options.

The regulatory and financial issues involved in designing new or updating existing health and care facilities will often constrain us into what we can do now by actually putting off what we should address in the long term. As a consequence we are not always aware of the bigger picture, and the greater issues of change that are constantly in play. This book therefore will attempt to break that circle, and provide a vision of how the current issues will affect our future.

Planning for future care is not a science but a combination of considered study of current trends together with an understanding of the past. It is not our intention to lay down a predicted future with any preconceived dogma, but because the stakes are high, it is our intention to offer information and inspiration as we plan today the type of health and care infrastructure which we will leave future generations to inherit in the 21st century.

Martin S. Valins
Derek Salter

Acknowledgements

The authors are particularly indebted to all of the individuals and organizations whose insights and visions form the core of this book. We thank them for giving up many hours of their time and offering highly practical and relevant information based upon their many years of experience in the field of health and care.

Many thanks to the following for their invaluable help:

All of the employees of Care Design Group, London, England and Baltimore, USA; Reese Lower Patrick & Scott, Lancaster USA; Salmon Speed Architects, London England; Mary Grauer, Hospice of Lancaster County, USA.

Special thanks to our respective partners and wives, Ginger Tippi and Jane Salter, for their love and support; to our parents, representing the generation that has handed down a legacy of experience and wisdom, Maisie and Hymie Valins and George and Marjorie Salter; also to Derek and Jane's children David and James, and to all children to whom we, in turn, must leave a legacy for them to grow and flourish.

Chapter 1
Looking Back

Martin S. Valins and Derek Salter

Introduction – historical overview

Originating in the time of the matriarchal goddess religions, when the cyclical process of nature and women's ability to give birth were revered, the relationship between the midwife and the woman giving birth was the first healer–patient relationship. It was a relationship of trust and equality in which two equals cooperated to bring life into the world. In primitive societies those seen as holding mystical powers came to acquire more formal ones. Thus healing and believing brought forth the faith healer. It has been said that within such an historical context it is possible to develop a rationale for the present situation and to produce a basis from which to appraise current trends and future directions.

Early knowledge was gained both from intuition, as well as from watching animals and then passing on accumulated knowledge down through the generations. Early healthcare took place in whatever environment was available. Apart from primitive tools there was no technology and medicine was based upon touch, comfort and belief.

The early Egyptians identified over 250 diseases and combined medicine with magic and religion. In *Unit 2000 – Patient Beds for the Future*, (Hamilton, 1993) Hamilton quotes Imhotep as being the first physician known to history dating back to 2300 BC. Coincidentally he was also an architect. As the Egyptians developed the science of medicine, treatments and drugs, there was parallel development in improvements to public hygiene and sanitation. Medical care however, if it did not take place in the home or community, was probably provided in temples as there were no hospitals at that time.

The Babylonians further developed medicine and records show that fees were charged for a healer's services. Yet it was the Greeks who gave us Hippocrates and the famous oath. Greek buildings used for medical care were still similar to temples. The Greeks however viewed healthcare in a natural and totally holistic framework. Their first buildings contained people who were in need of treatment and while they could be described as hospitals they were more akin to health resorts. Could this be where the word hospital, (i.e. a place of hospitality) originated? Dormitories were appended to these health resorts and the patients' dreams were interpreted by the priest. The Greeks assumed, as only natural, that healthcare treatment should include music, poetry, arts and good cuisine. The modern concept of alternative medicine is, paradoxically, traditional as it was the original and natural way of healing. The rise of 'technomedicine', chemical interventions and the concentration on parts of the body rather than dealing with the whole person, can therefore be reviewed as alternative.

From about 500 BC to 475 AD the Romans assimilated medical cultures from the territories that they inhabited. Generally, the Romans, as the Greeks, provided healthcare in the community. However, as a conquering nation, the Romans relied upon a healthy supply of slaves, gladiators and soldiers. They therefore built treatment centres for the enslaved or institutionalized. The Roman hospital was therefore based upon a military regime within a rigid institutional setting. Thus the early example of what has become known as the medical model was indeed based upon the military model, that is, the provision of care within an ordered and military setting.

The early Christian era, between 1 and 500 AD brought the return of women in the role of healers through the Church and convents. Hamilton quotes the first free Christian hospital as being founded in 390 AD.

During the chaos that followed the collapse of the Roman Empire between 500–1000 AD, monasteries retained the teachings of early Greek texts. Monks used their knowledge of medicine and herbs to care for the sick and the term hospital was still synonymous with offering hospitality, i.e., refuge from the ravages of the outside world.

Buildings for care were still built on a domestic scale. The exception was the Santo Spirito Hospital established by order of the Pope in 717 AD. The containment of a larger number of patients resulted in buildings which were similar in size and scale to religious institutions. As prayer was an important part of any treatment, so the larger care buildings resembled the Church aesthetic.

One can therefore begin to see how healthcare became detached from the spirit of healing in primitive societies and how the early teachings of Greek medicine were lost in the military and institutional settings of the Romans. Though healing environments offered by religious orders were spiritual in nature, the Church as an institution became the model for the building.

More scientific methods of healing appeared throughout the Renaissance period, 1400–1700 AD. This was also the time of Michelangelo and Leonardo da Vinci who saw, in true renaissance fashion, the integration of art, invention and medicine.

In England the traditional role of the Catholic Church in healing and medicine declined as Henry VIII broke away from Rome. Instead he encouraged and gave authority to physicians, granting the College of Physicians a charter in 1518.

Hamilton (1993) refers to the years 1550 to 1850 as 'the dark period for nursing'. Women were assigned nursing duty in lieu of a jail sentence. Many hospitals fell into decay, and insanitary conditions, epidemics and diseases were common. The hospital was seen as a place to warehouse the sick and dying and not necessarily a place for care and treatment.

It was not until the beginning of the Industrial Revolution that further advances were made in medical care. The hospital however, was still seen as a place for those without sufficient means to be cared for in their own homes. In the American colonies the first hospital was founded in Pennsylvania in 1751, with Benjamin Franklin as a Trustee.

Scientific and technological advances

The combination of further scientific study and epidemics such as cholera in the United States from 1830 to 1850 created a demand for more hospitals. As hospitals grew larger, so the incidence of cross-infection became greater. Florence Nightingale understood the need to plan care buildings to avoid cross-infection. She introduced a regime of greater cleanliness and order and the now famous Nightingale Ward, born out of the need for a stricter regime of care and discipline, left an indelible mark on the subsequent planning of healthcare buildings.

It is therefore interesting that both in the Crimean War and in the American Civil War, a need was recognized to improve medical care through cleanliness, discipline and scientific rationality. Treatment on the battlefield became the generator for new models of care planning. Surgery until then was always seen as a last resort. The outcome was invariably poor due to cross-infection and pain must have been horrendous without proper anaesthetic. Yet towards the end of the 19th century, with Louis Pasteur's and Joseph Lister's understanding of living organisms and methods of antiseptic, the surgeon came to the fore. As it became understood that surgery was best undertaken in antiseptic conditions, so the importance of the hospital as the focus of healthcare treatment became further established.

With the discoveries of X-Rays and radium, the diagnostic approach to healthcare became bound to a building rather than being brought to the people. Technological advances accelerated throughout the 20th century. Each bore the need for new equipment, with technology further centralizing and emphasizing the place of the hospital as the main focus of medical skills.

The present and the future

It is only comparatively recently that the focus has returned to care in the community. As medical invention and technology become further sophisticated so technology itself can begin to break away from hospital buildings and move into the community. Therefore the hospital no longer needs to be the focus of healthcare.

This is also reflected by the worldwide economic crisis in the funding of large hospital programmes and the enormous expense of hospital technology which encourages providers towards a low-tech form of treatment. Have we therefore come full circle? It may not simply be a matter of full circle, more that healthcare may have conceived the hospital mainly out of the necessity for quasi-military discipline and the need for improved cleanliness.

In the final analysis if we wish to view and envisage our future we have to return to the early and fundamental principles of the human condition. Perhaps the hospital was no more than an uninvited detour to satisfy a set of circumstances that may no longer apply. As will be seen in later chapters a major shift is now taking place away from the provision of large hospitals towards smaller satellite facilities that will be more accessible to local healthcare requirements. This change of emphasis reflects the universal need to reform and contain healthcare expenditure. In our post-industrialized societies, growing attention is now being paid to the concept of providing healthcare in the community.

0_____1800   2000_____2000+

Care takes place at home
    or in the Community

        Care takes place in Medical Institutions

                    Care takes place at home or in the
                                        Community

Fig. 1.1 Hospital, community home care.

As a reflection of these changes, opportunities are being created for new forms of buildings which will take the place of the traditional hospital and other centralized medical institutions.

References

Anon. (1993) Operation Health Care. *The New Republic*, **208**: 13; Issue 4080, March 29th.

Hamilton, D.K. (ed.) (1993) *Unit 2000. Patient Beds for the Future – A Nursing Unit Design Symposium*. Watkins Carter Hamilton, Texas.

Hoare, J. (1992) *Tide and Wave: New Technology in Medicine and the NHS*. (Report based on the proceedings of The Caversham Conference on Health Technology Assessment, 1992.) Kings Fund Centre, London.

Institute of Health Services Management (1992) *Europe and Health: Influence in the Centre. Proceedings of a conference held on the 13th March 1991*. Institute of Health Services Management, London.

Kings Fund Initiative (1992) *London Healthcare 2010: Changing the Future of Services in the Capital*. Kings Fund, London.

Murphy, E. (1992) *London Views. Three Essays in Health Care in the Capital*. Kings Fund London Initiative, London.

Robinson, R. (1990) *Competition in Health Care – A comparative analysis of UK plans and US experience*. Kings Fund Institute, London.

Sahl, R.J. (1986) The Hospital Changes in Building and Operation. Institute In Zusammenarbeit Mit Der Universität Düsseldorf, Düsseldorf.

Stocking, B. (1992) *Medical Advances: The Future Shape of Acute Services*. Kings Fund London Initiative, London.

Further Reading

Valins, L. (1993) *Intimate Matters: Restoring Balance and Harmony to the Feminine Experience*. Gaia Books Ltd, London.

Chapter 2
Healthcare Reform and Change

Martin S. Valins, Amy Reese and Ken Bast

Introduction

H.B. Gelatt, writing in *The Futurist* (1993) said that the future does not exist, never did, and never will. By definition, the future has not happened and when it does happen it becomes the present, and then quickly becomes the past.

An attempt to fathom how best we can envisage a future care landscape can become too complex and too parochial if we only pay attention to the particular mechanics and workings of various government systems within each post-industrial society.

The drive for change

The drive for change in healthcare delivery and availability by political means reached its zenith in the UK under the Labour government following the Second World War with the introduction of the National Health Service. Northern European countries have also developed universal healthcare systems. However, the closing decades of the twentieth century have been characterized by governments attempting to prop up systems based upon universal coverage, whilst at the same time it has been almost impossible for other post-industrialized countries such as the United States to introduce them. The failure in 1994 of the Clinton administration to push through a universal system of healthcare was testament to the fact that voters are cautious and reluctant to cast central government in the role of healthcare provider. Therefore we see a definite pattern emerging of governments moving away from being providers of healthcare to acting as regulators.

Whether for good or bad the market will be a major determinant of the type of healthcare delivery system which we can plan for in the future. The main factors affecting changes in long-term care may be summarized as follows:

- *Healthcare reform:* although perceived as a government legislative programme, reform is, in fact, already occurring from within, the drive being cost containment in the marketplace. Healthcare reform is about attempting to rein in the escalating costs of the nation's healthcare by offering a more integrated form of healthcare delivery.
- *Managed care:* healthcare will become increasingly 'managed'. The term 'case management' will increasingly be heard. It refers to the effective management of an individual throughout the continuum of the healthcare process; management being the operative word, implying forward thinking, evaluation and ongoing maintenance of that individual's needs. Case management should detect, anticipate and plan for an individual's needs to avoid unnecessary and often expensive healthcare emergencies or crises of intervention as a result of the system reacting too late in the process.
- *Day surgery:* because of advances in medical technology more acute hospital-related and medical treatments are taking place on a day basis. There is now less in-patient and more out-patient acute care. Hospital in-patient days have and will continue to be reduced.
- *Sub-acute care:* the earlier discharge of patients from hospitals is placing a high emphasis on home healthcare and the need for lower cost in-patient environments for recovery and rehabilitation where home healthcare is not an option. Such environments, referred to as 'sub-acute', are now increasing in number and will be in greater demand as hospitals look to offload their non-acute cases.
- *Specialist nursing homes:* in long-term care the nursing home is undergoing the same rationalization as the hospitals. Government subsidy programmes are seeking to control, by financial distinctiveness, shorter stays in skilled care. Patient assessment is encouraging nursing homes to attract high acuity patients and to seek to offload lower acuity (and by definition, less remunerative) long-term care residents into non-skilled environments such as assisted living or close care.

The consequence of the above is that if healthcare providers simply stood still and relied upon a traditional pool of consumers and services, occupancy levels and/or reimbursements would fail.

Change is also motivating varying levels of healthcare delivery to integrate and to co-operate. The concept of the free-standing healthcare building is over. Providers must become a part of a healthcare system network. In the healthcare delivery system of the future, a seamless continuum of care, void of walls and barriers will be the model. Alternative care settings will grow in type and size. This will involve providers aligning through ownership and other legal relationships to reduce costs, improve patients' outcomes, enhance provider viability and reduce administrative burdens.

In the past an integrated delivery system did not exist. Rather, care delivery was fragmented with no coordination between varying levels of free-standing health services. In the evolving healthcare delivery system, market forces are knocking down the old walls of fragmentation. The physical entity of a building or a site no longer defines the border of that facility's services. Providers must cross that border to find new territory in a managed care delivery system that is beginning to take shape, and which will provide opportunities such as

- linkages with hospitals/physician systems;
- contracting and alliances with payers – commercial insurance;
- subcontracts with multiple provider groups – hospitals, physician organizations;
- ability to prosper under different corporate arrangements.

What will future consumers be looking for?

Within the new paradigm of healthcare delivery even the word 'consumer' needs to be redefined. Traditionally, we would have perceived consumers primarily as patients who are receiving care. Yet the consumer may also be the contracting partner at the hospital, buying blocks of services on behalf of its patients. The network payer or provider may, therefore, become the consumer or purchaser of services with the patient or resident becoming the end user.

In terms of future demand and expectations, we will therefore need to examine the issues within three interrelated approaches

- scope of operation and services
- efficiency of operation and services
- quality of operation and services

Scope of operation and services

Within the emerging new systems of care, in reviewing the spectrum of services that future consumers will be looking for, there are many areas to be considered either as an enhancement of an existing service base or to broaden that particular spectrum. Several factors will place primary healthcare as an increasingly important focus towards the overall delivery of healthcare services. These may be summarized as follows:

Primary healthcare

The local physician or general practitioner working within the community is in the best position to 'manage' the care of his local patient population. As such the general practitioner can effectively and unobtrusively act as gatekeeper to other more specialized services.

Primary care can harness advanced information technology to ensure linkages with hospitals, consultants and availability of healthcare information not only from the region or from the country but on a global scale. Primary care can also utilize improved medical technology; certain surgical operations which would have required hospitalization can now be done on a day centre basis economically and effectively within a primary care setting.

Central to the role of primary healthcare will be the shift away from focusing upon treatment to prevention with ongoing health maintenance programmes related to diet, exercise and regular health check ups. So at a basic community level many of the more expensive surgical and chronic conditions may well be prevented by good health maintenance.

The primary healthcare model established as part of the UK National Health Service remains a model for many countries. In the United States the local physician as gatekeeper is now beginning to take on an increasing importance as health maintenance organizations (HMOs) see the primary healthcare frontier as an effective means of ensuring a more cost-effective healthcare delivery system.

The hospital

Fragmentation and specialization will be the key to hospital services of the future. A combination of the drive for more economic efficiencies, plus the sweeping changes which have occurred through the impact of technology render the large thousand bed hospital an anachronism in a future care landscape. As mentioned above many of the reasons why a person would have been admitted to a hospital are now becoming redundant as such procedures can be undertaken within a day in a primary care facility. Even when hospitalization is required, the duration of patients' stays is radically shortening. Both in the United Kingdom and the United States real estate agents have been trying to dispose of excess hospital land and buildings. As technology advances the downsizing of the hospital will be an increasingly evident trend. What remains of the hospital will be a high-tech hub where particularly expensive or specialized treatments that cannot be undertaken on a community or regional level will be delivered. As will be explained in Chapter 3 the move towards a more high-tech hospital environment does not necessarily imply a 'techno' building, devoid of sensitive and humane requirements. Indeed the hospital of the future, being part of a myriad healthcare alliances, will also need to harness our increasing awareness of the power of healing through the human spirit with more friendly and user-sensitive environments which involve nature, sunlight, massage, music, relaxation and alternative therapies.

Traditional skilled care

The provision of health and care services on a long-term care basis (2–3 years) primarily to older people (80+ years) has been the core of what is often referred to as traditional skilled care nursing services. While there will inevitably remain a segment of the population who require 24-hour skilled care, that core market is being challenged by the financial drive to push lower acuity level cases out into the community or into group housing or close care and assisted living programmes. Even for those high acuity residents, the system will not simply assume that high acuity equals long-term care. It is anticipated that patient stay, even within skilled nursing homes, will be reduced from the current average of 24 months to between 3 to 6 months. This challenges the very notion of long-term care within the skilled nursing environment.

Special care (Alzheimer's disease and related dementia)

Population data for most post-industrialized countries reflect a trend toward an increasing percentage of older people. With that top-heavy demographic shift comes a greater incidence of Alzheimer's and related dementia. Statistics indicate that the incidence of Alzheimer's disease increases with age, 5 per cent over 65, 20 per cent over 80. Although such cases require heavy care, their acuity state is not always high in terms of skilled care requirements. There will, however, inevitably be an increasing demand for innovative special care environments. Innovation and excellence will be prerequisites for attracting contracts with other neighbourhood healthcare providers for special care services, subject to reimbursement rates justifying the overhead of the care requirements.

Hospice care

Hospice and palliative care is a developing speciality in both the UK and USA. It focuses upon controlling pain and other symptoms, easing suffering and enhancing the life that remains. It integrates the psychological and spiritual aspects of care to enable patients to live out their lives with dignity, as well as offering support to families both during the patient's illness and their bereavement. The care provided by a hospice is developed specifically to meet the needs of the dying patient and his or her family. Specially trained staff are needed to control pain and other distressing symptoms and to give emotional support to patients and to their families.

The growth in hospice programmes in recent years has been considerable. While the desire to die at home is to be supported, this is not always possible. There are increasing incidents of people who are in the terminal phase of an illness who live alone, or where the carers themselves are unable to provide sufficient or adequate care and attention. Thus, there appears to be an increasing need for in-patient hospice programmes. The developing theme, however, is not necessarily to integrate these into a healthcare environment. Hospice providers view their programmes as quite distinct in terms of their culture of care and look to recreating the home rather than the healthcare facility within an in-patient hospice programme. The emerging trends in in-patient hospice care will need to be considered, as well as the financial viability with regard to the optimum number of beds to be provided.

Sub-acute care

Sub-acute care is increasingly gaining recognition as an important level of patient-focused care with considerable potential for cost savings. It is emerging so rapidly that by the year 2000 there may be a greater need for sub-acute care programmes than for any other level of care. Sub-acute care is making a real difference in the USA, not only in the quality of care to patients, but also in controlling rising healthcare costs. Sub-acute care is typically 25 per cent to 50 per cent less expensive than a similar acute care setting. The length of stay in a sub-acute centre averages between two weeks to six months. Many medically complex patients face

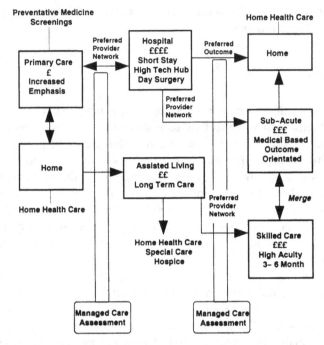

Fig. 2.1   Managed care: the implications for long-term care providers.

extensive periods of recovery. A less institutional physical environment is usually found in sub-acute care centres. To many the sub-acute arena represents a potential for nursing home providers. Yet, while there is potential demand for sub-acute beds, coupled with enhanced revenues, the sub-acute market may well become cluttered.

Assisted living/close care

Assisted living is now viewed as a long-term care alternative to the skilled care nursing home. It involves the delivery of professionally managed personal and healthcare services in a group setting which is residential in character and appearance and in ways that optimize the physical and psychological independence of residents. As case assessments and managed care continue to push the system down, so lower acuity level residents who would have normally resided in a skilled nursing home will be the future members of an expanded assisted living population.

Efficiency and operation of services

Cost containment and managed care will continue to be adopted as the mantras of the 1990s and beyond, so the efficiency of a healthcare facility becomes a critical factor in its survival. Both the marketplace and government want to see healthcare costs pushed down. Healthcare networks rely upon contracts with preferred providers who can demonstrate that they can offer quality services for a competitive price. Large payer groups such as managed care organizations will be able to negotiate from a position of strength based upon their ability to purchase beds and care in bulk.

In order to maintain the quality of care and the financial viability of a facility, overheads and non-productive expenditure will need to be scrutinized closely. This will include a re-evaluation of:

- administrative costs;
- care staff efficiency (number of working hours actually spent in the delivery of care, as opposed to administrative chores, meetings, etc);
- overhead costs of physical plant and food service delivery;
- energy consumption (lighting, heating, ventilation, air cooling etc.);
- maintenance of buildings in terms of systems, renewal/repair requirements of finishes and fittings;
- space utilization within the facility, percentage of building used for care versus administration – non-revenue producing areas.

Quality of operation and services

Despite the often diverse view of providers of healthcare facilities, there are some common threads about healthcare provision in the decades ahead. Without question, healthcare facilities of the future will offer a more consumer-friendly environment. Achieving that goal could take many forms, but in general it will be a move away from a medical institution towards a healing and therapeutic environment – a return to the Greek concept of 'hospitality'. Notwithstanding the financial pressures of providing effective healthcare environments, healing environmental design is less a function of money than of mindset. In many cases, construction costs are not significantly higher. The trend throughout the spectrum of healthcare is to move away from high-tech aspects of curing toward high-touch healing.

References

Cox, A. and Groves, P. (1990) *Hospitals and Health Care Facilities*. Butterworth Architecture, London.

Gelatt, H.B. (1993) Future sense: creating the future. *The Futurist* September–October.

Hamilton, D.K. (ed) (1993) *Unit 2000 –Patient Beds for the Future. A Nursing and Design Symposium*. Watkins Carter Hamilton, Texas.

Hamilton, K.S.A. (1993) *The Health Care Provider of the Future: a Strategic View of Health Care and a Successful Provider Response*. Hamilton KSA, Minneapolis.

Further Reading

Malkin, J. (1992) *Hospital Interior Architecture: Creating Healing Environments for Special Patient Populations*. Van Nostrand Reinhold, New York.

Miller, R.L. and Swensson, E.S. (1995) *New Directions in Hospital and Healthcare Facility Design*. McGraw Hill, New York.

Chapter 3
The Impact of Technology

Margaret Wylde and Martin S. Valins

Introduction

It would be difficult to overestimate the impact that technology already has and will continue to make in the future to healthcare providers and consumers. The impact of technology may be viewed within three distinct yet interrelated areas:

- medical technology
- information technology
- product design and supportive technology for end users.

Medical technology

The breakthrough in medical procedures such as the human heart transplant was not so much a result of improved technology as simply improved plumbing techniques by surgeons undertaking such procedures largely by hand.

Technology has however had an effect upon surgical procedures: for example the use of lasers for treatment, and the ability to use fibre optics to view and explore inside the patient prior to, during and after an operation. Technology associated with such procedures will become increasingly sophisticated, transportable and more cost-effective. This will lead to less invasive surgical procedures, which as previously explained, will often reduce the need for lengthy hospital stays for recuperation.

Technology is also advancing at a rapid pace beyond the surgeon's table as we begin to understand the miracle of the human being in terms of our genetic makeup. We have knowledge now that certain individuals with a particular genetic profile or heredity have propensities to some diseases. The term 'genetic engineering' is already on conference agendas and whatever moral, ethical or religious debate there may be, technology will exist in the very near future to alter an individual's profile genetically in order to prevent the onset of a disease. Perhaps this is where cures for cancer, AIDS, arthritis and Alzheimer's disease may be found. Perhaps there will even be a genetic cure for the common cold. Of course one can move into greater detail and read in awe of the technological advances that are being made across the laboratories of post-industrial countries. For the healthcare provider it could mean that diseases and conditions which now populate the wards and treatment centres of our health buildings may in time be cured perhaps by simple day surgery genetic reprogramming to banish today's major causes of death to medical history.

Information technology

Whilst medical technology is unravelling largely behind closed doors of laboratories, information technology is already an integrated and necessary part of our everyday lives. Personal computers continue to revolutionize basic administrative and office procedures. The Internet is helping to break down physical distances and make available information and data on a global scale. The information superhighway allows free form discussion between every user on the planet. Technology already exists for the country physician in West Yorkshire, England to converse directly via video conferencing with a top heart specialist in San Francisco. It is only a matter of time therefore before such technologies are introduced which enable a patient in the country practice in West Yorkshire to have access via his GP to the expertise of a worldwide medical community. Information technology itself quickens the pace of change and innovation. The more that we learn about information technology the more we can do. It is the sharing of information, the breakdown of physical barriers, instant access to expert advice, a databank of procedures, outcomes and alternatives, based upon an almost infinite resource which will at once allow medicine to be practised both more locally and globally.

Information technology and access to medical data is of course not only possible within the doctor's surgery but also within any person's home or community. Researchers at Kansai Science City in Japan have developed a notion of a high-tech smart house which includes a high-tech lavatory with equipment for measuring blood pressure and urinalysis. Such technology in the home or in the community may therefore even obviate the need for a visit to a medical centre. Instead, consultation, diagnosis and treatment could take place on the Internet.

High tech or high touch?

Technology however has a danger of being a 'Boy's Own' fascination. Our health is entwined with our relationship with each other, the planet and our wellbeing. Technology can only give us the means to a more effective and perhaps efficient method of improving our healthcare delivery systems. However, the possibility of societies of healthy high-tech hermits has to be guarded against.

Ancient healers relied on touch, massage, comfort and relaxation. Sigmund Freud showed how his talking therapy relieves much induced stress and mental phobias. Indeed it is a paradox that improved information access in many ways causes greater levels of stress in the workplace. In our faster paced lives we view solutions to healthcare as also needing to be intrinsically high-tech instant solutions. Healthcare maintenance and prevention is not only related to an improvement in diet and better exercise but into reducing unnatural or high levels of stress to avoid the need, or perceived need, for excessive use of alcohol or substance abuse. A gallstone may be cured now in a few seconds by a high-tech laser gun but stress caused by the breakdown in relationships both at home and in the workplace takes time, patience and understanding.

As post-industrial society continues to unravel, we must again recognize the need for centres of health to become places of healing. We need to reintroduce a sense of poetry, rhythm, peace and serenity in our inner souls and rediscover the healing powers of techniques such as yoga, aromatherapy or reflexology which can provide an alternative, or perhaps even a complement, to our high-tech future care. The health practitioners of the future, with their technical abilities now largely undertaken by computers, may need to return to the role of healer as portrayed in pre-industrialized society. That is, a healer who relies upon care, the good spirit and the touch and smile of an understanding and sensitive professional. The challenge of technology raises in turn this equally important challenge and reminder of our spiritual needs.

Product design and supportive technology

Where we were 20 years ago

Twenty years ago we thought of people who had differing abilities as completely different from ourselves, as being representative of an unfortunate event that would not happen to us. Today, despite the significant increase in the number of older people who have outlived the functional capacity of their human form, having a body which does not have the capacity it once had, this blinkered view still persists.

Twenty years ago, the attitude towards older adults was that their only option was eventually to take their place in a nearby nursing home. Assertive technologies which permitted individuals of differing abilities to deal with what would otherwise be hostile environments were few, functional and frightful. Most assisted technologies (which permit, or enhance use of another product) were developed to satisfy a specific problem and usually only addressed the singular function. Thus someone with differing abilities would most likely require a series of assertive products, each incompatible with the others and designed with little regard to the variations of human form or the environs in which they were to be used.

Where we are today

Although progress has been slow compared to the explosion of microprocessor-based devices, some advances have been made relative to products and technological design which better address the position of people with different abilities. This subject is best considered in terms of what we think (attitudes) and what we can do (behaviour).

Attitudes

What we think about people with different abilities is beginning to change. That is, we have begun to adjust our language and laws. First we recognize that speaking about the disabled, the elderly, the blind, the deaf, the wheelchair bound, robs an individual of his or her identity and classifies that person according to a physical, sensory or cognitive attribute. We recognize that discriminatory language did not recognize a person, nor differences among persons, but said that all persons who had problems negotiating environments, or who had reached a certain age were readily classified into a single group, such as the disabled or the elderly.

Several European countries and more recently the United States have passed legislation compelling businesses to ensure equal access to all prospective customers regardless of their abilities. Slowly changes have been seen in the design and construction of the commercial environment. Unfortunately, the changes and features designed to accommodate people of differing abilities continue to appear to be added on. That is, as an afterthought to the original design.

Today's accommodation of people with differing abilities continues to reflect the attitude that there is a dichotomy among the able and the less than able, or the young and the old. That is, it is only ever other people who require these accommodations and not ourselves.

Behaviour

Our attitudes are reflected in our behaviours, which are evident in the technologies that are available today. Few furnishings, fixtures and electrical items designed for residential environments incorporate universal design features that will enable people of differing abilities to use them. Most appliances, bathroom fixtures, electronics, components and furnishings are designed for the able-bodied market. Few offer features that would enable individuals with reduced physical, sensory or cognitive abilities to use them.

Many products for the home have added features and functions and have increased their complexity and reduced their usability by people who are less able. Indeed the electronics explosion has led mainly to manufacturers competing by adding feature after feature regardless of necessity or desirability. The goal is to boast of more features than our competitor, rather than of greater convenience, access and control.

Additional bathroom fixtures, some of the most challenging technologies in the residential environment, have not changed. Although changes in our abilities to use conventional bathing and toileting products are virtually inevitable, the design and function of such products have not reflected the fact that a greater proportion of the population is living longer.

There is an abundance of assisted devices for helping the bather or lavatory user, but most of these devices have an institutional or prosthetic appearance and are added on to the existing or ordinary fixture. Thus they are in the way of other users or they occupy space in rooms that are notoriously too small. Several companies have developed accessible bathing systems. While many of these products are easier to use than a traditional fixture, they are marketed as devices for the handicapped, have an institutional appearance, and have a price tag only affordable by a few.

Some rehabilitative technologies are, however, available that offer increased options and flexibility. One of the greatest limitations of the individual who uses a wheelchair is that of vertical reach. Retrieving items located at a height greater than 137 cm (54 inches) is almost impossible for most wheelchair users. Wheelchairs of today, however, are overcoming this problem. Several manufacturers offer manual wheelchairs that elevate the individual into a standing position and power wheelchairs that can raise and lower the seat.

With only a few exceptions however, other assisted technologies have changed little in their form or function since their advent two centuries ago. The majority of walking frames, canes and crutches in use today have the same appearance and construction as the earliest versions of these products. There are bright spots however. Changes in materials (graphite and aluminium) and the addition of features, options and even colours begin to recognize the difference and individuality of the people using the product.

Microprocessor-based technologies offer hope as we develop voice control, remote control, while increased capacity, speed and effortless software minimize differences among individuals. The lightning advancement of information highways and interconnection of people in remote places, the growth of telecommunication and the breadth of inactivity is likely to increase opportunities and reduce differences among individuals. Regardless of how one interfaces with a microprocessor device, the input (presentation) to the receiver is the same. The results achieved by someone who is blind, deaf or severely physically challenged will be comparable to all other users.

What is holding us back?

There are three primary circumstances that are holding us back. The first is attitude. The second is funding constraints. The third is lack of research.

The greatest challenge facing the improvements of technology in a future care landscape for less able people is posed by the prevailing mindsets among designers, builders, developers, manufacturers and the general populace. As long as the attitude is that it cannot happen to us, and that those who are differently abled are a small portion of the population, progress will be slow.

As the 'baby-boom' population looks around at themselves, and at their parents, attitudes are likely to change. As increasing numbers are involved in helping to find solutions caused by environments incompatible with the abilities of their ageing parents, a loud enough popular cry will be heard.

Agencies funding technologies for differently abled individuals are few. They fund products that meet minimum standards and solve problems encountered only by those with the greatest need. Because of these funding agency priorities, manufacturers are forced to focus on tasks and specific minimal solutions that are low cost. If on the other hand they were funded to improve products for the general populace, so that they would better serve people of differing abilities, the results would have broader acceptance and lower costs.

The third barrier to the improvement of technology is lack of appropriate research. Many companies lack in-house capabilities to understand the importance and benefits of consumer research. To many manufacturers research means a limited trial of a product by an in-house group of employees who have a vested interest in the design and development of the product.

Many technologies have had low acceptance rates by consumers because many inventors and manufacturers do not recognize that need does not equal want. People may desperately need a device to permit them to function independently but if the device does not reflect what they want they will go without rather than accepting something that undermines their self-image or sense of self-worth. Lack of research among the end users perpetuates lack of understanding and market dynamics.

Futurecare programme and planning requirements

Within the next twenty years we can anticipate changes in microprocessor-based technologies that we are not even dreaming about today. With linkages of communications and microprocessors and the laser-like intensity of competition among technology developers, performance standards of PCs are likely to change every two years – microprocessor-based technologies will have more than 1000 times the capabilities they have today.

Unfortunately the development of other technologies (furnishings, fixtures, appliances and home design) has not kept pace and continues to lag far behind that of the information superhighways. What good will the ability to stay at home be, due to improved communications, if we are prisoners imperilled by an incompatible environment? The number of people with differing abilities will continue to increase as the population continues to age and as high-tech medicine is increasingly capable of saving and prolonging life. Greater numbers of individuals are likely to have functional limitations as greater numbers survive longer and overcome illnesses.

The issues of the first decade of the 21st century will revolve around the problems encountered by ageing baby-boomers and the care they are providing to their parents. At that point the problem of incompatible development of information and supportive technologies will be felt keenly. Economics and information technologies will dictate that health care is administered at home but the inaccessibility of the home environment will create significant care giving burdens. Rather than being served by the advancement of information technologies, individuals and their families will be enslaved by them. Healthcare and health monitoring will occur at home but unless the concept of universal design is adopted, there will be few residential environments suitable for home healthcare.

The successful health and long-term care facilities of the future will outpace the residential environment in developing and incorporating technologies that enable individuals to maintain their independence. Because few homes will have furnishings and fixtures that will allow an individual to function independently, the residential environments that incorporate these features will be much sought after.

The immediate steps that must be taken in order to prepare and keep pace with information technologies of the future are for developers, designers and builders to embrace the diversity of human abilities in their educational programmes, language, products, technologies and environments. This recommendation does not mean the adoption of extant standards for barrier-free design. These standards represent minimal requirements and an infinite number of compromises. We

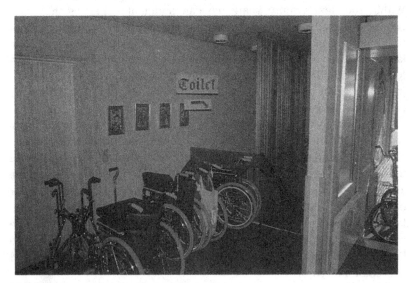

Fig. 3.1   Barrier-free design?

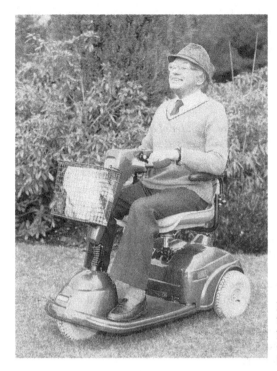

Fig. 3.2   Modern
technology can allow
patterns of living to
continue despite frailty.
(Photo: Sunrise Medical.)

should all strive to invest in serving the diversity of human needs with
the universally designed technologies that exceed their expectations in
quality and beauty. If the trend for technologies that serve people with
differing abilities continues on the track of meeting minimal standards
for special markets, both manufacturers and consumers will be losers.

The practical steps that need to be taken now are:

- For a language of universal design to be developed that does not
  incorporate minimal standards but that focuses upon principles that
  embrace the diversity among individuals.
- For research to be undertaken to define human self-sufficiency needs
  and to understand the impact of self-image, self-worth and wants.
- For developers, architects and interior designers to recognise how
  perilously far behind the information technology wave they are and
  how quickly they must refocus design and development of products
  for people of differing abilities.

If we are able to recognize the potential which technological advance
offers in terms of future care environments, we should not squander that

opportunity by approaching it in the same blinkered frame of mind which has persisted for so many years. We are capable of radical vision, and the opportunity to fulfil it must not be wasted.

References

Hamilton K.S.A. (1993) *The Health Care Provider of the Future: A Strategic View of Health Care and a Successful Provider's Response*. Hamilton KSA, Minneapolis.

Further Reading

Branson, G.D. (1991) *The Complete Guide to Barrier Free Housing: Convenient Living for the Elderly and Physically Handicapped*. Betterway Publications, Crozet, VA, USA.

King's Fund Commission (1992) *London Health Care 2010: Changing the Future of Services in the Capital*. King's Fund London Initiative, London.

Leibrock, C. and Behar, S. (1993) *Beautiful Barrier-free: A Visual Guide to Accessibility*. Van Nostrand Reinhold, New York.

Pirkl, J.J. (1994) *Transgenerational Design: Products for an Aging Population*. Van Nostrand Reinhold, New York.

Stocking, B. (1992) *Medical Advances: The Future Shape of Acute Services*. King's Fund London Initiative, London.

Chapter 4
Primary Care

Martin S. Valins

Introduction

The two great professions of medicine and architecture both have their own proud histories of achievement, scientific and technical advances and the overwhelming desire to improve the wellbeing of the human experience. The interface between the two, occurring in buildings designed to accommodate and facilitate the practice of medicine can therefore generate a dynamic fusion in the pursuance of professional excellence. History has taught us, however, that it can also lead us to the clash of two established cultures.

During the later part of the 19th century and for the majority of the 20th century, it was the hospital which became firmly established as the main focus of medical skills and has therefore been the focal point of dialogue between architecture and medicine. Nevertheless in a post-industrial society, growing attention is now being paid to the concept of providing health care in the community. Architecture for primary healthcare is therefore an increasingly important issue which involves aspects of both medicine and architecture.

What is primary care?

Primary healthcare may be described as a nation's first line of defence in maintaining the health and wellbeing of its people. Its services are often the first (primary) contact a patient has with the health services system. Additional facilities may perhaps be provided for hospital consultants to hold outpatients sessions within a local health centre. Other organizations such as self-help groups, family therapy and child guidance may also occasionally use such a centre. Primary care can therefore be defined as all those services provided outside a hospital by family doctors, dentists, retail pharmacists, opticians and other

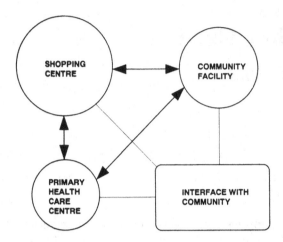

Fig. 4.1   Primary care facility as part of a community resource.

healthcare professionals allied to healthcare working in a community setting.

Health care at the crossroads

On analysis of the many healthcare systems throughout the world, there is evidence of a change in emphasis away from the provision of large hospitals towards smaller satellite facilities situated within local communities. This is in response to the almost universal economic crisis in funding large hospital programmes and has coincided with advances in technologies of healthcare and preventative medicine. However the economic arguments for reducing capital and revenue expenditure in hospitals can only be sustained if there is first the establishment of an adequate infrastructure of such community-based primary care facilities. These economic and technological factors have also influenced the recognition that there are social and medical benefits for patients in taking services such as non-acute and outpatient care out of hospitals and into the communities. For example, in the United Kingdom the concept of healthcare in the community has been embraced by successive governments, largely perhaps for its apparent economic savings of public expenditure on centralized resources.

As a reflection of these changes, opportunities have been created for new forms of buildings for primary healthcare. It has also created an opportunity for a new format of dialogue between contemporary medicine and architecture in a community-based context.

Smaller community-based facilities allow for a greater integration and identification within the local community. They can offer an improved access and availability of medical care, incorporating the needs and requirements of the patient as a local user/resident. Many of the activities within such a centre will largely depend upon patients accepting the invitations to attend, for example, preventative medicine programmes. Such programmes will therefore stand a better chance of success in an environment designed to be accessible, welcoming and comfortable.

New design parameters

Primary care centres therefore offer both medical and architectural practitioners the chance to break away from the often negative images of the hospital. At worst these were typified by the 19th century hospital building which arguably was not much improved on during the construction programmes of the 1960s. Because of its sheer size and scale, it became almost a cathedral of medicine. Patients and junior staff would pass in awe through the enormous corridors where unfamiliar smells reinforced a sense of alienation from the medical staff. Despite (or even because of) often chronic underfunding in the public sector many such hospitals remain (with some loss of dignity) inappropriate environments for the delivery of health care. In some instances when located on a hospital campus, primary care centres can form a bridge between the community and the services of the hospital on a more human scale.

Innovation and radical change have been most prominent in primary healthcare programmes in the United Kingdom. Currently primary healthcare in the United Kingdom is delivered from a variety of premises ranging from converted shop units and doctors' own homes, to multi-purpose built primary care facilities. It is only recently that primary healthcare services have come to occupy their prominent position in the general field of debate on health policy.

The changing face of primary care

Primary care has traditionally been a service which has suffered from a lack of co-ordination among the various paymasters of primary healthcare practitioners, from independent contractors which include general practitioners, dentists and opticians, to the salaried community health staff which include district nurses and health visitors to salaried local authority staff which include social workers.

Since the 1980s the greater emphasis on primary healthcare has also been linked with consumerism, accountability and value for money. Furthermore in an attempt to improve coordination between the various bodies involved in primary healthcare, major organizational shifts have taken place in both planning and management.

Since the mid 1980s as a part of the reorganisation in UK primary health care, many Family Health Services Authorities (FHSAs), which now administer the services of general practitioners, dentists and opticians, undertake surveys of existing practice premises, particularly in the inner cities, to gauge overall existing standards and to encourage, where possible, improvements. As a result of these surveys FHSAs have become better equipped to plan and identify the required services and premises in collaboration with other Health Authorities, with particular regard to immunization, vaccination and child health surveillance.

A further debate, concerning primary healthcare services and its problem of narrow definition, was set out in the 1987 White Paper, *Promoting Better Health: The Government's Programme for improving Primary Health Care* (HMSO, 1987). Early discharge from hospitals as part of the move to managed care will increase the current trend towards continuing care in the community for patients with chronic disorders provided by general practitioners and their health staff. In the United States and Scandinavia, this is beginning to lead to community-based facilities specifically serving patients which function as resource centres for primary care.

The new organizational changes will respond to the change in demands for primary care. In the United Kingdom hospitals undertake day surgery and reduce the length of stay in acute wards. In addition, the

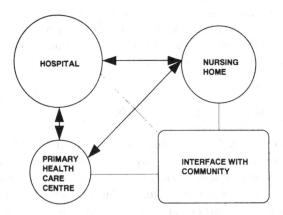

Fig. 4.2 Primary health care facility as part of a medical park.

government is promoting a greater emphasis on the provision of care in the community rather than centralized institutions for patients with long-term disabilities. This also implies that the increasing number of older people will require long-term support to be provided in the community rather than in institutions. All this, combined with a general view that primary healthcare facilities are the most appropriate vehicle for preventative health programmes, will bring the services and facilities of primary healthcare into greater focus in the future.

The key objectives of the new government programmes in primary health care are as follows:

- to make services more responsible to the consumer
- to raise standards of care
- to promote health and prevent illness
- to give patients the widest range of choice in obtaining high quality primary care services
- to improve value for money
- to enable clarification of priorities.

Each of these will imply better standards of building for the delivery of primary care. In particular the Family Health Services Authorities are being encouraged to play a more active role in administration and planning of such services and facilities including

- setting the targets for preventative services
- inspecting and monitoring standards of premises
- provision of more comprehensive information on practices services
- the listing of public comments on the quality of those services provided.

In 1990 a new contract of service for general practitioners in the UK was introduced, and the following year the most major change in the way that GPs were structured came into being with the concept of fund holding, whereby practices of at least 11 000 patients were offered the opportunity to be given a fixed budget of primary and secondary care in order to:

- improve the quality of GP services
- help GPs develop their practices for patients' benefits
- give GPs greater control over the use of resources
- encourage hospitals to be more responsive to the needs of GPs and their patients.

The minimum requirement has since dropped to 9000 patients with further programmes expected to allow practices of 4500 patients to become eligible as fund holders. The intended benefits of fund holding are reduced hospital waiting lists, greater communication and cooperation between consultants and GPs, and reduced costs.

The future of primary care

Primary healthcare is not an unequivocal concept. It can be interpreted from either a functional or organizational point of view. Most of the tasks of primary care in the majority of western European countries are dealt with by private practitioners. In many of these countries, such as Great Britain, Ireland, the Netherlands, Austria and Denmark, primary care is controlled through political decisions concerning those countries' health services.

In the future an increasing number of nurses will be trained to be able to perform more of the tasks that have hitherto been carried out by doctors. In Canada and the United States, for example, nurses can already undergo specialist training to become nurse practitioners. A similar development will take place in the United Kingdom, particularly in medical screening and health information with certain categories of nurses performing increasingly independent and more qualified tasks. All these rely upon suitable building environments in which to allow such progress and change to happen.

Managed care places a particular emphasis upon effective primary care services. Primary physicians will need to be allied to managed care networks in order to attract future patient groups. In turn, general practitioners are now being encouraged to promote their healthcare services and in effect compete within the newly created marketplace of primary healthcare. Managed care will also encourage a broader range of services including the undertaking of minor surgical procedures. This will no doubt benefit the patient and remove the pressure for services from hospitals; however, the undertaking of such procedures will rely upon adequate and appropriate facilities. If the managed care group demands these services, so the provision of appropriate environments will need to respond to these demands. In an attempt to exert greater financial control over the cost of primary healthcare, general practitioners will be increasingly asked by both public and private payers to be more accountable in the running of their primary healthcare services. Although the financial independence of general practitioners has been jealously guarded, there will be a trend towards larger groupings of primary physicians contracting with managed care organizations. Para-doxically the increased job security of contracting, perhaps as an employee of a managed care group, may attract more physicians to enter general practice, at a time when liability insurance and other practice overheads are deterring many from doing so.

The above factors will shape and influence the type of buildings needed to accommodate a future primary healthcare service. Good architecture becomes a marketing tool and the public face of an efficient and well organized primary healthcare centre.

In the United Kingdom, while the underlying trend is to improve premises, greater control is being exercised by the government over the amount of available funds. From 1990 budgets for general practitioner practices became cash limited. Notwithstanding the radical change in the country's economic fortunes, it appears unlikely that the strict controls of capital expenditure budgets will relax significantly under different political regimes. Such capital underfunding will force general practitioners to explore alternative forms of financing, better premises or simply to delay the building projects until state funding becomes available.

The Tomlinson Report into the UK National Health Service which was published in 1992 endeavoured to address several of these issues, and caused enormous protest by actually advocating the closure of several London hospitals and the amalgamation of others, in order to redirect available healthcare resources into a greater and enhanced programme of community-based primary care.

Global trends

Primary health care will become the major vehicle for the delivery of healthcare services particularly in inner cities where family structures and problems of extreme poverty are reaching a critical stage.

The poor nations of the world, caught in a vicious circle of malnutrition and disease are, of course, in urgent need of aid and support. The concept of primary care as a community-based and essentially low-tech infrastructure for health promotion and illness prevention will prove the most appropriate framework of support than the import of westernized medicine and technology within hospitals.

Supporting primary healthcare facilities will allow appropriate and indigenous technology and medical expertise to develop, respecting the autonomy of culture as an integral part of health care. There is much that the communities of the world can learn from each other.

The death of an individual from hunger is a tragedy repeated far too often throughout the continent of Africa and parts of Asia. Yet there is also the tragedy of an unnecessary death caused by the failure of a person's heart due to excessive cholesterol and high fat food. It is within such extremes of world affluence and poverty that primary healthcare will play an increasingly important role for future generations.

While attention and financial resources are quite rightly required in Third World countries, there are also the inhabitants of the Fourth World. These are the deprived and run-down inner city areas of often quite prosperous First World centres. Primary community care in major cities such as London, Birmingham, Washington DC and New York etc., suffers from a current lack of medical staff and facilities. The debate still rings out loudly about the need or otherwise for large and perhaps now outdated hospitals in these areas and is expected to continue for some time. The provision of adequate facilities will therefore continue to be a major problem on the future care landscape. Yet within the inner cities there is limited land on which to build. Even when sites are identified they are prohibitively expensive. Further hurdles are sometimes erected by insensitive planning or zoning authorities.

It is here perhaps, where people are most in need of even the most basic and fundamental healthcare services, that we lay down the gauntlet of challenge for a future care that can provide adequate preventative health programmes.

Care and treatment facilities

In order to attempt to break the vicious circle of urban and Third World blight, it is here perhaps that future care becomes inextricably linked with finance. The world is full of possibilities, subject to the consumer wanting or being able to afford new and exciting services. Future care is about the wonder and possibilities of a techno-medical world where the technological superhighway performs dazzling miracles with ingenious equipment, with laser precision.

Yet how does this help the single parent family, starved of sufficient basic primary healthcare services? How do we hold the mirror of the new technology possibilities of tomorrow to the young infant dying of malnutrition or disease simply because its mother's milk was not sufficient? Only improved primary healthcare services can begin to answer these incredibly complex questions. That is the challenge for futurecare.

References

Alford, T.W. (1979) *Facility Planning, Design & Construction of Rural Health Centres.* Ballinger Publishing Company, Cambridge, Mass.

Beales, J.G. (1978) *Sick Health Centres.* Putman Medical, London.

Bosker, G. (1987) Architecture as an asset in health care. *Architecture,* **January**, 48–53.

Bryant, J.H. *et al* (1976) *Community Hospitals and Primary Care.* Ballinger Publishing Company, Cambridge, Mass.

Cammoc, R. (1981) *Primary Health Care Buildings.* The Architectural Press, London.

Conference of Missionary Societies (1975) *A Model Health Centre* (working party report by 1972 Medical Committee) Conference of Missionary Societies in Great Britain and Ireland, London.

Cox, A. and Groves, P. (1990) *Hospitals and Health Care Facilities.* Butterworth Architecture, London.

Davies, C. (1988) Architecture of caring. *The Architectural Review,* **1096**, 15–17.

Dudley Hunt, W. (1960) Hospital, clinics and health centers. *Architectural Record.* F W Dodge Corporation.

Gaskie, M. (1985) Re-inventing the hospital. *Architectural Record* October 1985, F W Dodge Corporation.

Goldsmith, S. (1984) *Designing for the Disabled.* RIBA Publications, London.

HMSO (1987) *Promoting Better Health: The Government's Programme for Improving Primary Health Care.* HMSO, London.

Hannay, P. and Hallett, K. (1987) Doctors on the street and preventative medicine. *The Architects Journal,* **186** (**38**), 127–132.

Havlicek, P.L. (1985) *Medical Groups in the USA 1984.* American Medical Association, Chicago.

Hoglund, J.D. (1985) *Housing the Elderly.* Van Nostrand Reinhold, New York.

International Union of Architects Public Health Group (1989) *Reference and background paper of the UIA-PHG to WHO-DSHS District Health Systems.* 26th April 1989.

Knight, C. III (1987) Designing for the health care process and market place. *Architecture,* **76(1)**, 48–52.

Malkin, J. (1982) *The Design of Medical and Dental Facilities.* Van Nostrand Reinhold, New York.

Malkin, J. (1990) *Medical and Dental Space Planning for the 1990s.* Van Nostrand Reinhold, New York.

Marks, L. (1987) *Primary Health Care on the Agenda: A Discussion Document.* King's Fund Institute, London.

Marks, L. (1988) *Promoting Better Health: An Analysis of the Government's Programme for Improving Primary Health Care.* King's Fund Institute, London.

Paine, L.H.W. and Siem Tjam, F. (1988) *Hospitals and the Health Care Revolution.* World Health Organisation, Geneva.

Pearce, I.H. and Crocker, L.H. (1985) *The Peckham Experiment: A Study of Living Structure of Society.* Scottish Academic Press, Edinburgh.

Pritchard, P. (1981) *Manual of Primary Health Care.* (2nd edn.) Oxford University Press, Oxford.

Redstone, L.G. (ed.) (1978) Hospital and Health Care Facilities. In *Architectural Record.* McGraw-Hill Book Company, New York.

Reizenstein Carpman, J. *et al* (1986) *Design that Cares* American Hospital Publishing Inc., Washington DC.

Robinson, R. (1990) *Competition and Health Care: A Comparative Analysis of UK Plans and US Experience.* King's Fund Institute, London.

Rostenberg, B. (1987) *Design Planning for Free-standing Ambulatory Care Facilities.* American Hospital Association, Chicago.

Sahl, R.J. (1986) *Das Krankenhaus: Wanglungen in Anlange und Betrieb.* Deutsches Krankenhausinstitut, Germany. No **94** March. (German Hospital Institute in Co-operation with the University of Dusseldorf.)

Seliger, M. (1986) *Health for all in Finland.* Laakintohallitus ja Teki jat, Tampere.

The Swedish Planning and Rationalization Institute of the Health and Social Services (SPRI) (1984) *Primary Health Care in Progress.* SPRI, Stockholm.

Stallibrass, A. (1989) *Being Me and Also Us: Lessons from the Peckham Experiment.* Scottish Academic Press, Edinburgh.

Stone, P. (1980) *British Hospital and Health Care Buildings.* Architectural Press, London.

Valins, M. (1975) *Community Health Centres.* North East Thames Regional Health Authority, London.

Valins, M. (1990) *Surgery Design Update 1990.* MV&A Research, London.

Valins, M. (1993) *Primary Health Care Centres.* Longman Press UK in association with John Wiley & Sons Inc.

World Health Organisation (1985) *Targets for Health for All: Targets in Support for the European Strategy for Health and for All.* World Health Organisation Regional Office for Europe, Copenhagen.

Chapter 5
Community Care in The United Kingdom

Deirdre Wynne-Harley

Introduction

The tradition of community care has a long, diverse and fragmented history. From the early days of monastic care and alms-houses forms of care and support have been offered in or by communities for those who were frail or incapable of self support. The 1834 Poor Law saw the beginning of the central regulation of Poor Law institutions – the workhouses for able-bodied sane adults and specialist institutions for others. The groups in need of segregated care were identified as children, the sick, the insane, the defective and those who were aged and infirm. It was not until the period after the Second World War that the moral arguments against segregation were strongly and widely voiced. A pamphlet *50,000 Outside the Law* published by the National Council for Civil Liberties (NCCL, 1951), highlighted the plight of those '... who while certified remain a race apart outside the protection of the law'.

The second half of the 20th century has seen a search for a definition and formulation of an integrated policy for care in the community and for community care. In 1957 The Royal Commission on the Law Relating to Mental Illness and Mental Deficiency (HMSO, 1957) stressed the need for a move away from hospital and institutional care, declaring that it was in the best interests of patients who are fit to live in the community that they should be enabled to do so, and that local authorities should assume responsibility for those who were not in need of in-patient care. This report provided a basis for the Mental Health Act of 1959.

Looking back, it is evident that the focus of debate and much legislation was centred on aspects of mental health because of the dual role of the state in both the provision of care and in providing protection for the community by the removal of threatening people. Fear of people with 'disordered minds' still remains an inhibiting factor, influencing attitudes towards policies of integration and community care for people leaving psychiatric hospitals and for those with learning disabilities.

The first community care plans were formulated in 1963 when local authorities were asked to assess and report on the expected needs of their populations and their current levels of service. The reports which followed highlighted the very wide variations in provision between authorities, even those with social and geographical similarities. From this time onwards the ideal of community care found a broad consensus, whilst the issues of practice have given rise to political and philosophical conflict.

During the 1970s changes were made in local authority organization, bringing together a number of departments providing personal care and welfare under one umbrella as Social Services Departments (SSD). This resulted in a much sharper divide between health and welfare services; on the one hand it clarified their roles whilst on the other it created a new need for greater coordination and cooperation between the two. It must be noted that frail elderly people were, and are, those whose needs continue to be most at risk of neglect when coordination is inadequate.

Recent developments

Despite the ostensible lead role of the SSDs in providing formal services, during the 1980s there was a rapid growth of informal, voluntary and private sector care and government policy was directed towards a 'mixed economy of care'. Thus during this period private sector residential care in particular received a great boost through a system by which residential and nursing home fees were met in full by the Department of Health and Social Security. As a result the number of places for older people and those with physical and mental disabilities nearly doubled between 1979 and 1984 (the exact figure was 97 per cent). Whilst the government policy of encouraging the commercial sector remained firm, the anomaly of doing so through public sector expenditure could not continue and in April 1985 the DHS acted to impose national limits. Nevertheless this form of subsidy still represents a major source of income for private homes.

The 1980s saw a major expansion in the need for care, particularly among very elderly people. This, combined with economic pressures and the ideological commitment of the Thatcher government, shifted the emphasis from care in the community provided in the main by local authorities to private care by the community in the home or in residential settings. The burden thereby fell increasingly upon family and friends as costs of private care rose, exceeding levels of available statutory support.

Issues of today

The themes of the ideals of community care for the past three decades or so are still present, and these include

- the belief in the rights and dignity of persons in need of care
- the belief that people prefer to be cared for in their own homes, or in settings which are homelike and on a domestic scale
- the belief that individuals in need of care should have choice and influence over the care they receive.

Of these ideals the value placed upon individual choice is perhaps that upon which the greatest theoretical myths have been founded. The idea of choice is central to the White Paper *Caring for People: Community Care in the Next Decade and Beyond* (HMSO, 1989) and yet even if we accept the constraints of the proviso 'within available resources', the goals of value for money and efficient case management coupled with the emphasis on non-state provision immediately inhibit any effective cross-sector choice for the user. There may indeed be less choice than before implementation of the Community Care Act. For example there are few, if any, instances where an elderly person assessed as being in need of residential care is able to make a choice of home from either private, voluntary (non-profit making) or statutory sector, unless they are able to fund themselves. The 'level playing field' recommended in the Griffiths Report between public, voluntary and private sector residential care was firmly rejected when residents in non-statutory homes were granted income support and housing benefit subsidies, thus giving financial incentives to local authorities to purchase beds in the independent sector rather than retain their own residential establishments. People who are assessed as needing residential care are thus being prevented from exercising any realistic choice.

The assessment process

The assessment process is the key which unlocks the door to community care, and yet assessment is a long way from provision which is the meeting of individual needs. It would be unrealistic to disregard the very real economic pressures under which many authorities work and to underestimate the problems of allocating scarce resources. However the present 'contract culture' appears to limit user influence and increase that of the purchasing professional, largely on the basis of which needs

Health care expenditure expressed as percentage of gross national profit (GNP)

1987 figures	% GNP	Compared with average of OECD countries (8.4%)	Percentage change 1977–87	Compared with average percentage change in OECD countries (18%)
Denmark	6.7	–1.7	–8	–26
Finland	6.7	–1.7	–3	–21
Japan	5.2	–3.2	+2	–16
Sweden	8.9	–0.5	+7	–11
UK	5.8	–2.6	+12	–6
USA	11.1	+2.7	+25	+7

Health care expenditure in £ per person (1987)

	Health care expenditure	Compared with average of OECD countries (885)	Percentage change 1977–87	Compared with OECD average change (+60%)
Denmark	777	–208	–4	–64
Finland	732	–153	+31	–33
Japan	625	–260	+189	+120
Sweden	1002	+117	–5	–65
UK	423	–462	+41	–19
USA	1252	+367	+51	–19

Fig. 5.1   Health care expenditure per capita and as a percentage of GNP in 1987 (source: International Monetary Fund).

can be realistically met. At the beginning of 1995 an appeal procedure was set up for users or their supporters who wish to contest a professional assessment. The effectiveness and influence of this will be carefully monitored, particularly by agencies who work with older people and those who have disabilities. It is undoubtedly a potentially valuable tool for consumers and their carers.

Funding shortfalls

At the time of writing – mid 1990s – we are at a critical point, possibly a point of no return in the provision of social welfare. The local authorities' role as providers of direct services has been minimized to the extent of offering little more than a safety net or last resort service. The undermining of publicly funded residential care in particular, has reached a stage where many authorities have maintained only the barest minimum of beds necessary to cope with emergencies. This wholesale abandonment of traditional areas of care has not only reduced user choice but has also threatened to recreate the scenario of past years when the institution was a last resort. Public provision is not only being reduced, but by being starved of funds and by the loss of the stimulus of being a place of choice, its buildings are also in danger of being run down and neglected possibly beyond a point of no return. There are also dangers to the voluntary sector, which in the past possessed many centres of innovation and excellence. Within the climate of competitive tendering, financial pressures will limit the scope and flexibility with which such agencies have maintained their autonomy and supported their client groups.

Community care based on a commercial model – a supermarket style consumerism – carries an inherent threat to public welfare provision. As with glossy advertising the suggestion is planted that if a product is on the shelves, choice is assured and the consumer will have access to the goods of their choice. What then of the frail and vulnerable people in need of care but unable to shop around and with no realistic say in the matter?

Does the community care?

Community care is not only a matter of availability and distribution of resources. Above all it depends on attitudes prevailing in society itself. The community in many ways sets its own agenda for care. One clear indicator is its willingness or otherwise to welcome projects in its own neighbourhood. The 'not in my back yard' (NIMBY) principle unfortunately applies all too often, as when the majority of planning applications for accommodation for people with learning disabilities or those leaving psychiatric units are contested at every stage by local residents.

Future prospects

To consider the future of community care from the perspective of today is dismal. The tasks are how to undo past mistakes, to seek out answers which will provide the models for the next century and to ensure that training will meet new needs and challenges – these tasks face the policy makers and planners now and they should not be hijacked or diverted by politicians or subverted by the dogmas of fashionable theories.

We know the numbers of people over retirement age who will be in the population in the first decades of the coming century (barring massive natural or man-made accident). In brief, the number of older people (over 65) will increase until 2041 at which point numbers will begin to decrease. Within this age group the percentage of people over 85, after a sharp drop in the second decade of the century, will rise to over 15 per cent in 2051 (OPCS 1983). What cannot be predicted is the proportion of the total population these figures represent because that depends upon the birth rate which shifts unpredictably according to changing social circumstances and attitudes.

In the context of known figures certain assumptions and estimates have been made. For example, if the present figure for dementia (one in five over age 85) is maintained, by 2021 some quarter of a million old people will be affected and in 2041 that figure will have risen to more than 300 000. Other official statistics also raise anxieties for the future. For example, it is the population aged over 80 who rely far more on the health and social services than do younger age groups. They have more home visits from general practitioners and form the bulk of the case-loads of district nurses. Domiciliary and day care services are largely used by old people, as are an increasing number of hospital beds.

Are the right conclusions being drawn from the statistics and should planners follow the herd? Professor Margot Jeffreys (1987) challenged 'predictions' of increases in the extent of disability among survivors in old age. She states that:

Populations

	Population 1990 (million)	% of population aged 65+	Population estimated 2020 (million)	% of population aged 65+
Denmark	5.12	15.4	4.80	21.2
Finland	4.97	13.0	5.04	19.9
Japan	123.87	11.4	132.61	20.8
Sweden	8.31	17.7	7.82	21.8
UK	56.19	15.6	56.08	17.8
USA	248.43	12.2	304.36	15.4

Fig. 5.2 Demographic trends into the twenty-first century (source: *Compendium of Health Statistics* (1989), 7th edn, Office of Health Economics, London).

... advances in medicine and improvements in living conditions have enabled many who at previous times would not have survived ... to live on, perhaps with some disability into their seventh, eighth and ninth decades. ... But those who see this as a threat also ignore other contemporary changes which will affect the future pattern of health among the elderly. For example, medical advances have not only enabled the very disabled to survive into old age; they have also reduced the future dependency on others of very many elderly people ... thinking here of hip replacements and coronary by-passes.

She could also have added the removal of cataracts and cornea replacements to the list of surgical procedures which enable or enhance independence.

Evidence suggests that the 'young old' today are in general better off and in better physical and mental health than the previous generations at the same age. It seems probable therefore that in their older years this trend will continue and their health will be better than that of today's 80 and 90 year olds.

Practical issues in future planning of community care must not be distorted by negative thinking or fear of what might be. A search for positive approaches and flexible solutions should be the overreaching concern. However, community care is not based only on the delivery of services or the adaptation of accommodation. It has much to do with the whole environment in which we live and how the community feels about itself and upon the values placed upon its members, their needs and different stages of life.

It is easy to cite a set of guidelines such as the 'ideals' quoted earlier. These may be developed thus:

- Any form of care must preserve and when possible enhance the dignity and individuality of the recipient.
- Care should be available where the user wishes it to be.
- Care should be given in a manner and environment which is aesthetically acceptable to the recipient.
- Care should adapt to changing needs and wishes of the recipient.
- Both formal and informal care should reflect these guidelines.

It follows that user/consumer involvement in individual care planning should be a continuing process, but also that forward planning should be encouraged in earlier years to ensure a suitable home environment. For example the design of 'retirement housing' especially in private sector developments is often woefully inadequate, making only small concessions towards creating an environment which supports and facilitates continuing independence and in no way addressing future needs satisfactorily. Cost is frequently cited as a factor although this is seen to be a feeble excuse in the light of the excellent schemes produced on tight budgets by some housing associations. There is also new thinking in the field of flexible 'lifetime' housing.

Rapid changes in medical techniques have brought massive increases in the incidence of day surgery, in turn raising the possibility of similar increases in mobile surgical teams extending the potential of the hospital-at-home. Whilst new homes should not seek to emulate a clinical environment there are aspects of this new type of service delivery which should be addressed within the overall consideration of how people can best be assisted to maintain independence and autonomy in their chosen environment.

Conclusion

This chapter has attempted to show that whilst community care has a long history in the UK, it has been a history of inequalities and mismatch of theory and practice. Understanding and recognition of needs has not ensured that there were satisfactory, effective or acceptable ways in which these needs were met. The chapter has also sought to demonstrate some of the fallacies behind the negative attitudes which influence past and present policies and to encourage a positive approach to future care.

References

HMSO (1957) *Royal Commission on the Law Relating to Mental Illness and Mental Deficiency (The Percy Report)*. Her Majesty's Stationery Office, London.

HMSO (1989) *Caring for People: Community Care in the Next Decade and Beyond (The Griffiths Report)*. Her Majesty's Stationery Office, London.

Jeffreys, M. (1987) *An Ageing Britain: What is its future?* Centre for Policy on Ageing, London.

NCCL (1951) *50,000 Outside the Law*. National Council for Civil Liberties, London.

OPCS (1983) *Population Projections by Government Actuaries: Principal Project 1983–2023*. Series 13. Her Majesty's Stationery Office, London.

Chapter 6
Outcomes in the Environment – Long-term Care

William Russell

Introduction

When one looks to the future of care for frail and dependent people it is imperative to develop an accurate perspective on the current situation. The features that currently define long-term care are impairments in cognition and mobility. These two factors account for the permanent placement of the vast majority of patients in nursing homes. Our greatest gains in the care of these people will come through optimizing the environment and care giving that will change the image of chronic illness during the next 20 years.

The developed nations benefit from the major advances in healthcare accumulated over several centuries. Sanitation, personal and public hygiene, nutrition, education, immunizations and breakthroughs in some infectious diseases account for the reasonable expectation of a full life which most people experience. The reality is that medical technology has yet to make the most significant contribution to that process. In fact when the frailty of old age is contemplated it is often the burden of medical technology that is most feared. There is a perception that old age often includes a phase of dependency with an associated suffering and loss of control. This perception is further reinforced by the current state of housing, care giving and public policy concerning the chronically ill.

A new way of thinking

The fact that medical technology has a poor track record in the area of chronic illness is no surprise. It reflects the limitations that illnesses with slow progression place on researchers who must demonstrate results within a matter of months to compete for funding and complete fellowships successfully. The problems are long-term, and so should the efforts at solving them be.

The great breakthroughs in chronic illness will eventually come from people who make it their career to study a given illness and through dramatic advances in genetics and molecular biology. Those advances will benefit future generations of people but there are already so many people in society destined to develop chronic illness such as Alzheimer's disease, osteo-arthritis, cerebrovascular disease and other debilitating conditions that defy cure, that it makes a discussion on the factors that determine the burden of these illnesses germane. Yet it is in this arena that our greatest triumphs will come.

The manifestations of chronic illness

In general there are four factors that determine the manifestations of chronic illness

- the intrinsic realities of the disease
- the host
- the environment
- the level of care.

While any new treatments that may arrive will be welcomed, it should be assumed that a magic bullet of cure lies beyond futurecare. Dementia may be seen as an example although the same concepts can be advanced for any condition that produces frailty, vulnerability or dependency.

In the absence of a cure the most common therapeutic goals are to maximize function and avoid discomfort. Just as in pain management, the same treatment that prevents pain might prove ineffective in the relief of active pain, so in dependency, preempted manoeuvres to limit disability will be the most effective.

Disease factors may be the least amenable to intervention. In the case of dementia, the affliction may be latent for many years even before the onset of any awareness of the illness. It is often most tragic in disorders of cognition that the victim is not fully aware of the disease. It is often the family that will seek medical evaluation. However, it is within the areas of both care giving and appropriate physical environments that there seems to be the greatest promise for enhancing the life of people afflicted with chronic illnesses. Experience has shown us that when one of the major determinants of illness destabilizes a function and it is lost it is very difficult to regain and recover. In contrast to the current psychiatric dictum with regard to Alzheimer's disease, a positive development in one domain could render a wider benefit. Simply stated, the slow inexorable decline commonly associated with dementia is often a result of dysfunctional care environments and can be ameliorated or even reversed by improvements both in care and the surroundings in which it is provided. This is a reflection of the trauma of placement itself, a process that is inappropriately delayed, sometimes generated by inadequate housing or care giver burn-out and all too often by medical misadventures such as inappropriate procedures or therapeutics.

It is the goal of supportive programmes and nursing homes to reaffirm dignity, independence and self respect. The implications of this approach are that basic functions such as toileting, eating and walking are to be encouraged and restored. When such basic needs are met in an appropriate way it is common to see those gains serve as a springboard for additional improvement. People who were once tube fed can be retrained to eat and ultimately to feed themselves. People who are dangerous in their own houses because of wandering off or other issues in home safety can come to recognize their own space and belongings through more appropriate settings and so regain their independence. They are enabled to develop a sense of being safe and secure that supersedes many of the anxious moments they had when living in the community.

Implications for the future

We are at a time of enormous change in the expectations surrounding long-term care. We are breaking down many of the self-limiting beliefs about nursing home residents. As a result, we no longer require residents to leave hope at the door. As our understanding of the relationship between the environment and good health become better understood and as care giving techniques that emphasize comfort and function replace inappropriate medical regimes so we will begin to see a change in the natural history of chronic illness.

When one views the problem of chronic illness from a demographic perspective, one sees that in a given population at risk there is a percentage of people who are diseased, a percentage who may well be asymptomatic, a percentage who are functionally impaired, and a percentage who have died. While life expectancy has increased, the number of people, particularly women, who are experiencing disability in their final years is increasing. Excess disability will accelerate the symptomatic phase of illness and increase the rate of decline.

The greatest challenge for the future will be to develop, and make affordable, housing and services that are supportive and respectful of the elderly. At the same time, there must be a change in attitudes towards chronic illness. Public policy makers and health care providers must have a full realization about the nature and prognosis of disability. Early detection is important in contrast to the medical dictum that says if you don't have effective therapy then what is the point of making a diagnosis. The fact is that optimal housing and care giving are therapy in themselves.

People are better able to make decisions about housing and tolerate relocation early in an illness than later on. With effective case management and appropriate individualized therapeutics we can accomplish ageing in place avoiding the disabling experiences of serial placements and acute hospitalizations. Our goal must be to reduce excess disability and improve quality of life. When host or disease factors cause decompensation then the restoration of function will be the norm and not the exception.

The other part of the necessary equation is an improvement in the perspective of health care providers about the limitations of technology and the burdens associated with its indiscriminate use. We place a very special and vulnerable segment of our society at risk of needless pain and suffering. We may occasionally prolong life only to prolong suffering. We must proceed cautiously here however with healthy respect for the gift of life. When we then couple rational use of technology with the sophisticated union of services and settings we will see that chronic illness becomes a very different experience for the chronically ill person and for the people who care for them. In addition the proportion of people who arrive at a terminal stage of the condition will be greatly reduced.

The future of caring for the infirm, frail and vulnerable members of humanity can be an affirmation of the values that have been forged by a thousand generations of love and a reverence for the aged. In the words of Leo Tolstoy, 'It is not in caring for oneself that man lives but in caring for one another.'

We therefore must challenge the expectations and potential of medical technology to deliver the cure all approach. While life expectancy will no doubt increase, how can this be balanced both ethically and morally against the issues of the quality of life? Rates of disability and dependency may well increase as more people survive into old age. We must view the need for long-term care as a consequence of poor housing, health education and care giving during the earlier stages of life and as with any form of healthcare delivery, it cannot be seen in isolation. If we do, long-term care may ultimately pick up the bill for inadequacies in the overall healthcare delivery system.

Chapter 7
Senior Day Care

Joe Jordan

Introduction

Senior centres, as they are known in the USA, are community centres for older people providing a special place to spend leisure time in social, recreational and educational pursuits while offering a convenient connection to a network of services for elderly people. Their original purpose was simply to provide older people with socially enriching experiences to help preserve their dignity and enhance their feelings of self worth. Today they offer a significant range of social and supportive services to the individual through their professional staff and often become the focal point in a community for the delivery of these services. It is estimated that 15 per cent to 20 per cent of elderly people participate in their activities.

In many respects senior centres are homogeneous, especially in the concept of offering group activities and individual services, management and staffing by a few professionals, augmented by a larger number of volunteers and dependent on public funding to finance their operations and capital improvements. Variations from the norm are most likely to be found in facility size, operating budget and extensive programme services and activities that are available to the members. Not surprisingly these three characteristics of size, budget and programme offering are interrelated.

While senior centre facilities vary considerably in size the average centre has a floor area of only 5000 square feet and accommodates 100 participants daily. Larger centres with floor areas of 15000 to 30000 square feet are uncommon (probably under 10 per cent of the total) but can provide for 200–300 people or more on a given day. These are often referred to as multi-purpose senior centres. Most often located in larger metropolitan areas and small cities. They have increased staff, rely less on volunteers, are better funded and provide a more sophisticated array of programming options.

The first senior centre in the United States opened in New York in 1943. Their early development was an outgrowth of the senior citizen clubs that came to life following the Second World War and paralleled the break up of the traditional family structure and the emergence of the nuclear family which provides no accommodation for the grandparent generation. Where the senior clubs were mostly grass root, volunteer support groups that came together weekly for social activities, senior centres evolved from the leadership of charitable and religious organizations, joined later by financial assistance or sponsorship by local government. With paid staff and a governing board of directors they set out to provide supervised group activities on a daily basis. During the 1950s and 1960s they expanded throughout the United States and by 1975 their number had grown to 2500.

Looking back 20 years

To understand the changes that senior centres have undergone during the last two decades it is useful to look at the developments in public health and government policy that have shaped these changes. The passage of the Older Americans Act in 1965 was an acknowledgement of and a response to problems being experienced by rapidly increasing older populations. Through giant leaps forward in medical research and treatment the lifespan of Americans was being dramatically extended. Many were retiring at a younger age and living to an older age. Man's age-old dream of a longer life was finally being realized.

But the old dream brought new realities and new problems. The discomfort and limitations of declining health took their toll with ageing. Retirement savings had to last longer, as inflation ate away at fixed income. With advancing years some saw their lives as less satisfying. For many, social contacts were seriously reduced by retirement, loss of health or death of intimate friends and by the moving away of their children and neighbours. Some found themselves experiencing periods of depression or becoming socially and sometimes even personally inactive.

Alleviating many of these problems had been the original goal of senior centres. They provided a new social context where older people could associate with their peers, form new friendships and fulfil their social, physical and intellectual needs. Funds from the Older Americans Act 1973 amendments had a profound influence on their growth. They became a logical location for the act's congregate meals programme which provided a nutritious daily lunch in a group setting for little or no cost to the participants. The daily meal became the attraction that brought more members to the centres and involved them in a rich programme of activities that could now be scheduled around the lunch period.

The most impressive change over the past 20 years has been the explosive growth in the number of senior centres. During three decades before 1975 their count reached 2500 but in the following two decades the number had multiplied to 10 000, a four-fold increase. This growth was spurred on by grants and technical assistance from the local and state area agencies on ageing (Triple As) that had been established in the Older Americans Act. A tremendous boost came from the Nutritional Institute of Senior Centres (NISC). A programme of the privately grant funded National Council on the Ageing (NCOA) was created to conduct research and establish standards to guide the development of these new community facilities.

At the beginning of this period the principal change in programme focus for senior centres was a strengthening in the delivery of individual social services. Facilities which had been planned for a variety of group activities found themselves short on private office space for the case workers and administrators who were needed to oversee an expansion of government grants for social services which required extensive record keeping.

The early centres operated largely out of space borrowed from other social institutions but since the mid 1970s the picture has reversed and 75 per cent of the centres now have their own stand-alone facility. The average size has increased from 5000 to 7500 square feet and the number of those attending the typical centre has doubled from 50 to 100. The early stimulus of federal funding has decreased and the budget shortfall has been helped with some addition of state, county and local dollars while private support is up by over 35 per cent. Staff size at an average centre has more than doubled but dependents and volunteers have remained steady at a ratio of five volunteers to each paid staff member.

The demographic profile of centre participants has changed somewhat with the largest percentage increase occurring in those who are 75 and older. This is matched by a corresponding reduction in the percentage of those who are 65 and under. Racial and gender mixes remain unchanged: 85 per cent white, 11 per cent Afro American, 3 per cent Hispanic, 75 per cent female to 25 per cent male. Not surprisingly we find a 35 per cent decrease in health status and a 58 per cent increase in those considered to be frail.

Senior centres have become a mature institution. The types of activities and services offered at one centre are not likely to differ too much from those at another. A recent study based on responses from over 400 centres reports that the number and types of activities and services offered reveal little change over the past seven years.

Looking ahead: the next 20 years

The task of tracing the development of senior centres over the past several decades has been simplified by a wealth of data provided through three research surveys that have been conducted at seven year intervals. Centres have gone through a gradual process of growth and maturity with few surprises or major turning points. The senior centre has become an accepted American institution with a clearly defined role – its basic characteristics are unlikely to undergo significant change in the near future.

In all probability the incredible advances in medical science will continue at or beyond the astonishing pace that has been set over the past decade. Few doubt the predictions of longer life spans and the corresponding growth in the elderly population. At the minimum a matching increase in the number and size of senior centres can be expected. The prospect of other changes is much less certain.

This uncertainty is tied to the public policy in the field of healthcare and social welfare, both of which are currently under intense debate in the United States. However, since the elderly population has long been recognized as one of the most powerful lobbying groups, it is likely that legislative outcomes will favour them with greater assistance and benefits than they have at present. In order to achieve a greater potential of service, senior centres will require an increase in public funding.

One of the ways that senior centres will expand in the future is through the dynamic process of mergers and consolidations. In response to past increases in their level of funding urban multi-purpose senior centres have grown by establishing satellite facilities to deliver services and make activities available to individual neighbourhoods in various parts of the metropolitan region. A logical outgrowth of this approach will be the uniting of existing agencies and management groups to combine their resources and form networks of centres that may be able to serve the larger community population better, at a reduced cost. Such an increase in efficiency in coverage will be encouraged by federal and other public funding policy.

In addition to these changes in size, organization and management, there exist considerable opportunities for programme expansion beyond the array of activities and services that we have come to expect at a centre. Some of these are already under way but all are likely to become more prevalent in the decades ahead.

The administration for ageing has been encouraging centres to provide services that may be characterized by the term 'Eldercare' which addressed the needs of persons at risk of losing their independence. This includes those of very advanced age, individuals with lower incomes and persons with minority backgrounds. Among this vulnerable group are many without close family members to turn to for assistance. Eldercare services may involve transportation assistance, adult day care programmes and activities that deal with racial, cultural or language differences. Their goal is to help this group continue to maintain their lifestyle of relative independence.

In contrast to Eldercare which provides assistance in a group setting at the senior centre, community based care offers help to older persons in their own homes where they can receive periodic assistance in the activities of daily living. Since most people prefer to remain at home, even if this means staying with relatives or in a foster home, senior centres with a strong outreach programme can provide the meals, friendly visiting and special assistance that the essentially home bound person may require. Such in-home services enable the senior centre to offer continuous care to those who do not require an institutional setting.

Senior centres have long seen themselves as the community focal point for the delivery of services to the elderly. Indeed they have been encouraged to assume that role by the Federal Administration on Ageing. The concept in its ideal form is to house all ageing services at a single location and to offer a one-stop shopping opportunity where all forms of assistance may be obtained. Since specialized aid is offered by different private and public agencies each with its independent management and staff, the senior centre's best option is to offer rental space within the centre to those specialists on a part- or full-time basis. The advantages to the service providers are better communication with their peers, direct and easy access to their constituents and a more efficient operation.

As centres increase their efforts to help the more frail and at risk elderly, they may decide to join the growing number of sponsors of assisted living facilities. When the time comes that some are no longer able to provide for their daily needs without some regular help from others, this type of housing can be a more appropriate alternative to the traditional nursing home. The development and provision of assisted living by senior centres is still uncommon because of the heavy financial burden involved.

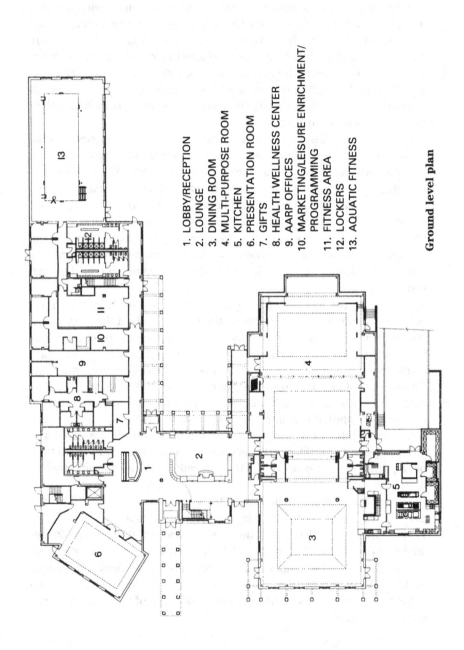

1. LOBBY/RECEPTION
2. LOUNGE
3. DINING ROOM
4. MULTI-PURPOSE ROOM
5. KITCHEN
6. PRESENTATION ROOM
7. GIFTS
8. HEALTH WELLNESS CENTER
9. AARP OFFICES
10. MARKETING/LEISURE ENRICHMENT/
    PROGRAMMING
11. FITNESS AREA
12. LOCKERS
13. AQUATIC FITNESS

Ground level plan

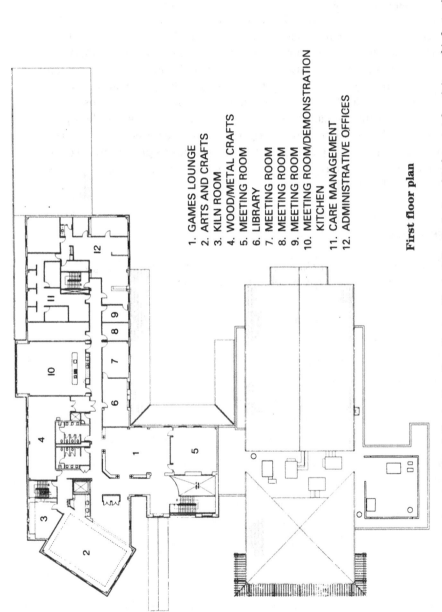

1. GAMES LOUNGE
2. ARTS AND CRAFTS
3. KILN ROOM
4. WOOD/METAL CRAFTS
5. MEETING ROOM
6. LIBRARY
7. MEETING ROOM
8. MEETING ROOM
9. MEETING ROOM
10. MEETING ROOM/DEMONSTRATION
    KITCHEN
11. CARE MANAGEMENT
12. ADMINISTRATIVE OFFICES

First floor plan

Figs 7.1 and 7.2 Burnham Brook Senior Day Care Centre. The building is designed to be a total activity and information centre for older adults. Architects: Wallace Roberts & Todd Battle Creek MI.

A more readily achievable form of housing assistance can be the referral to, or development of, foster home care. Foster care for elderly people is not unlike the familiar foster care for children. A family provides a home and the immediate services and assistance that the older guest requires in exchange for a monthly payment. This living arrangement offers special dividends in personal freedom, loving care and a degree of independence that cannot be found in a nursing home where regimentation and impersonal care are usually the rule. In summary we can expect senior centres to continue their traditional role of providing services and activities to 20 per cent of the older population and to increase in size and numbers through mergers and consolidations. Their most significant change in the coming years will be to widen their programme offerings to the frail elderly, provide space for other agencies to increase direct services in specialized fields and to play a more active role in satisfying elderly housing needs through assisted living initiatives and direct home care.

Reference

Jordan, J.J. (1979) *Senior Center Design: An Architect's Discussion of Facility Planning*. National Council on Ageing, Washington DC.

Chapter 8
Life Care – Looking Back Today, Future Programming

Robert Dana Chellis

Life care may be defined as an integrated managed care continuum of housing for older people embracing support services, social programmes, health care and health insurance.

Looking back

Thirty years ago major retirement homes in the United States operated under non-profit sponsorship. Minimal public funding was available for housing for the elderly with or without services. Then occupancy of traditional homes for older people dropped rapidly despite population growth. Sponsors were forced to recognize that education and higher expectation demanded more service-orientated housing for the elderly with privacy and control of one's life and activities. This process continues today. As non-profit homes serve more than the totally impoverished, 'give them what they need' has given way to 'give them what they want'.

In America, the Social Security Act in 1935, Hill-Burton Funding of Hospitals after the Second World War, Medicare and Medicaid in the mid 1960s, HUDS (Housing and Urban Development) financing programmes, and many other government initiatives and interventions have artificially channelled the growth of most retirement housing and healthcare since the days of the new deal. Life care however is one market category, a combination of housing, services, health care and health insurance – which has pursued a steady and demand related evolution.

There have always been isolated, multi-level housing and health related communities, but examples of modern life care programmes began to multiply in the 1960s notably in Pennsylvania, California, Florida and parts of the mid-West. Most of these early programmes were church related, all were non-profit making or in partnership with non-profit making organizations and the best were widely admired and imitated.

Launched by non-profit making organizations and largely funded from residents' home equity, scores of life care programmes opened. They offered socially rewarding, independent lifestyles with meal and many other services and on-site nursing care covered by an entry payment plus a monthly fee. All early sponsors offering life care had to self-insure the cost of nursing care for residents because neither good actual information or any insurance company products were available until the 1980s. Only non-profit making providers accepted the risk of self-insuring. Entering the 1980s, over 98 per cent of life care communities were still in the non-profit sector.

During the 1980s life care's growth potential was recognized by more developers, this time profit making bodies. Innovations increased. Units continued to get larger and amenities more notable. Entry fees became larger but more often refundable. By 1986 a few insurance companies began offering group life care policies encouraging for-profit developers to move from continuing care (i.e. without a 'lifetime contract') into life care. Many developers affiliated with non-profit making sponsors for the purposes of image building and greater marketability. Many non-profit making organizations retained commercial ones for development or management services. This surge of interest including Marriott Hotels' announcement of their plan to develop 150 facilities in 5 years was stifled in the recession of 1990–1993. Banks virtually stopped lending, bond underwriters raised their requirements, potential residents struggled to sell homes, states began regulating life care more tightly and growth was severely curtailed. Much discussed as this product is, growth to date is estimated at less than 1000 life care or continuing care communities serving less than 1 per cent of the over-65 market. Strikingly some isolated markets have penetration rates approaching 20 per cent, generally where a number of attractive projects meet an educated or an affluent market.

The issues today

After recession setbacks in the early 1990s, many new life care proposals are for smaller projects. This simplifies zoning (planning) approvals, reduces risk, eases financing and minimizes expensive pre-marketing construction and occupancy periods. Although they lack some economies of scale, having fewer amenities and services, and often lacking on-site nursing beds, new projects with fewer than 100 units are being planned more often than the previous 200 or 300 units. Thus the scale of life care which was originally considered too large for European, and particularly United Kingdom markets, has now been reduced in size and scale. Therefore the concept of life care becomes a form of community care which may be feasible even bearing in mind the more restrictive sites and planning regulations in the United Kingdom.

In the United States the industry remains fragmented and local, with only a few major players. As units become smaller, life care projects become more varied, more affordable and more likely to offer alternative payment options.

It is startling how quickly momentum lost by the life care industry has been seized by the assisted living industry. Assisted living is a form of long-term care housing with care services and meal provision. In the United Kingdom it may be equated to very sheltered housing. In the United States, assisted living is often loosely regulated, reflecting the desire of government agencies to offer alternatives to in-patient programmes. Some assisted living facilities market themselves as less costly than nursing homes, others stress the preservation of independence. For many people, such services do make nursing home care unnecessary.

Life care attracts active older people with an average age of 76–9. Typically in residence for 10 to 14 years they will never be impoverished by nursing costs or forced to leave. Assisted living projects however attract residents in their 80s with stays averaging 1.5 years to 4 years. The insecurity of a traumatic move to an unfamiliar and expensive off-site nursing home may be demanded just when the resident is at their most frail and vulnerable. In the United Kingdom this is overcome somewhat by the concept of close care. Essentially, close care consists of a number of self-contained apartments or cottages which are unobtrusively situated on the same campus as a skilled nursing facility. Both the apartments and the nursing home remain financially autonomous but at least there is the comfort of the availability of services either in or from the skilled nursing facility for the residents in their apartments.

Education is the key to preparing the elderly for increasingly long years of retirement. If they wait until they are unable to care for their house, their poor health may preclude a move to life care, leaving assisted living as their most viable option. They and their families must struggle to determine the best solution. Sponsors and developers should help educate the public to the real issues and adjust their products to meet evolving need as well as demand.

Future programming and planning requirements

Where will we be in 20 years? Even when joining or creating networks for greater efficiency home care agencies will be strained to the limit by

the sheer numbers of the elderly. Near universal insurance coverage will
further encourage unchecked demand for home healthcare services. In
the United States nursing beds will be in short supply after years of
restriction on construction to restrain runaway health costs. Assisted
living facilities will be built in large numbers by the for-profit sector.
Some, hastily planned and built, will struggle with low occupancies.
Others which become fully booked will be severely strained by residents
who have become heavy care users whilst in residence. Once in assisted
living many residents who are already in a process of declining functional abilities will strain staff capabilities. While resisting increased fees
to cover their heavier care, the shortage of nursing beds will make
transfers difficult. Education and greater awareness of alternatives
should increase the demand for life care generating long waiting lists for
limited spaces. But life care will remain in short supply due to the difficulty in raising initial funding, achieving complex approvals and
reaching high pre-sale levels for unbuilt programmes.

In the United States health insurance will become nearly universal
with simplified and almost universal billing systems, but the whole
system will still struggle to cope with demand and control costs. Many
facilities will be overwhelmed by the demands of empowered and
insured elderly people in their area. Delays in care delivery will decrease
and dissatisfaction will encourage a new tier of expensive private paid
clinics, nursing homes, hospitals and alternative medical centres.

While life care remains a privately financed alternative it should be in
a strong market position. Care coordination in such an on-site continuum offers the best assurance of effective health outcomes for life
care residents. While this mirrors the national trend towards managed
care networks, it requires no government financing. Life care meets
health care and support service needs and offers a healthy mix of social,
recreational and educational activity. For some it offers the most personal reward of their life.

Life care at home or life care without walls also has potential.
Embryonic in the early 1990s, it is a form of managed care ready to
blossom in the new environment. Life care at home offers coordination
of prepaid health and services to residents still in their homes, where
most prefer to remain. Early programmes, expensive and with few
benefits until care was needed have been slow to reach the market.
However, if life care at home can be wrapped around a life care campus
with immediate access to all the club-like social, recreational, educational amenities, and dining, plus health clubs and fitness centres, the
residents can access all this in addition to gaining insurance for home
care and nursing costs. If the US government finally mandates long-term

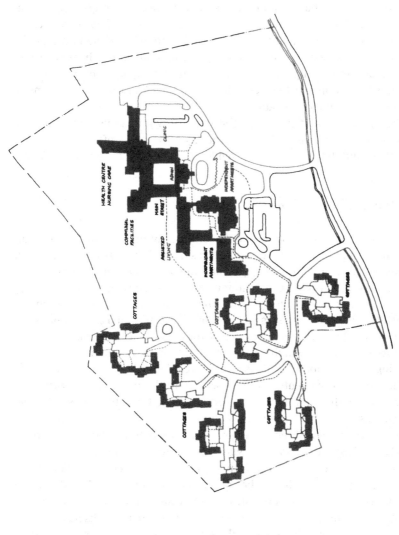

Fig. 8.1 Carleton-Willard Lifecare Village, Massachusetts USA.

care insurance, this will simply lower the cost and broaden the market for this product. This may strengthen life care centres and life care at home may become a major success in its own right. This could be a pleasant surprise for the private sector in the future.

Sponsorship diversity may prove to be another surprise as colleges, affinity groups and other constituencies sponsor their own retirement centres. College based life care takes advantage of the growing enthusiasm for life-long learning. Other groups like musicians and trade unionists may approach sponsorship in the tradition of medieval guilds, taking care of their own. Retirement programmes which involve fostering apprenticeships, master classes and acting as mentor for young people may compensate in a small way for the deteriorating situations of families and public education.

The challenges of the early 21st century will include high insurance costs, greatly increased demand, scarcity of trained staff and home care workers and the pressures to provide expanded but affordable services.

Solving the problems

The appearance of 21st century facilities may not be dramatically different, though many will look more residential than institutional. Even when research urges change, typical sponsors, directors and others, who commission and use most buildings are conservative in their development outlook. Direction by committee further stifles innovation and a fresh approach. Many users are reassured by traditional appearances but important changes may occur below the surface. Technology will bring 'smart' capabilities which will be wired into more and more new houses during construction. Buildings will self-regulate with greater and greater efficiency and residents will have access to the expanding information highway, with every kind of information at their fingertips. Medical diagnosis will be no further than an interactive computer and computers will be typical amenities. Emergency call systems will become increasingly wireless, often with two-way voice communication.

To realize the potential of future facilities, we need to challenge our sponsoring and planning bodies and project executives. They should be aware of the literature, innovations and evaluations and success stories. Sponsor committees should visit outstanding sites and discuss options with users and operators. Carefully selected development teams must be pressed to produce handsome, high-level and effective products. Great designs owe as much to enlightened sponsors as to great architects.

While every generation of the elderly arrives with higher expectations, education and observation may make more of them realize that more independence is achieved by pooling their resources with others than by clinging to their own real estate. Life care can offer greatly enhanced security, many more social, educational and recreational opportunities, all supportive services available as needed, companionship, and even insurance for health care risks. No other product covers retirement, physical, financial and psycho-social needs so completely or is so well positioned to grow in the next decade. Public awareness of the alternatives is the key to growth.

Reference

Chellis, R.D. (1992) *Lifecare.* Lexington Books, Lexington MA.

Chapter 9
Close Care and Assisted Living

Martin S. Valins and Gregory J. Scott

Introduction

At best it is a person's right to remain where they wish until they die. No doubt the majority of people would prefer to stay in their own homes, but with the onset of the consequences of ageing certain daily tasks of living can both inhibit and isolate a person from taking an active part in the community. While healthcare at home can bring a diverse and increasingly technologically sophisticated service into a person's home, this could still result in that person becoming a high-tech hermit. The need to live within a supportive and caring environment will always attract a significant proportion of our elderly population.

In our review of future trends in health care, two building types seem destined for an uncertain future. These are first the hospital, which will turn increasingly towards a form of high-tech hub, networked with satellite treatment centres within the community. The second building type is the nursing home.

The nursing home

The nursing home evolved out of the hospital. Geriatric wings of hospitals were traditionally the environments where elderly people too frail to maintain an independent lifestyle were warehoused within essentially institutional and medical settings. Chapter 10 discusses how the traditional nursing home model is likely to disappear from a future care landscape within the short rather than the medium term. This chapter deals with the alternatives.

As the nursing home becomes increasingly viewed as an inappropriate setting, so too have attempts to market so called independent housing for retired people floundered due to the developers' insensitivity to the needs of the consumer.

Sheltered or independent retirement housing

Post occupancy evaluations indicate that 'independent' or 'sheltered' forms of housing for seniors has tended not to take account of the consequences of the ageing process or as it is referred to 'ageing in place'. The issues that occur are linked to both the physical design (accessibility) as well as residents placing an increasing demand upon care services as their needs grow and become more complex over time.

Two factors have caused major problems in both the marketing and management of independent housing. The first cause is that the average age of entry into independent housing has been rising steadily over the past 15 years. We are reaching our retirement years healthier than before, and the services of home healthcare prompt many people to delay the move to retirement housing until the onset of some form of apprehension or incident relating to their health. By the time, therefore, a person seeks retirement housing, they may already be in need of assistance with the activities of daily living.

The second cause has been a basic lack of sensitivity by providers and architects as to the inevitability of ageing in place. A resident population of a newly completed independent retirement complex may be, say, in the 75 to 80 age range. Ten years on that same group of residents will be 85 to 90 years. This places an increasing demand upon care services to be provided by the management companies who also need to operate within a building framework that may not have been designed to cope with the inevitability of an ageing resident population. Marketing units, as they become vacant over time also becomes difficult as the average age of the resident population in say 5 to 10 years is no longer the 75 to 80 age band that the marketing was originally aimed at. It is a phenomenon unique to housing for elderly people.

The underlying problem with defining housing types by age is their lack of flexibility both in terms of their physical design and management services. Ideally all housing should be designed to cope with a range of age types and disabilities. However, even within 20 years this may not be achieved. A more achievable goal is to view and act on the recent developments in close care or assisted living. Close care, as previously described, comprises either cottages or apartments specifically designed for older persons but self-contained. They are built unobtrusively close to points of healthcare, i.e. a nursing home or a care base. Assisted living is similar in concept although there are many examples where they are not so deliberately linked to healthcare components.

Assisted living and close care – possible solutions

Regnier (1994) defines assisted living as a 'long term care alternative which involves the delivery of professionally managed personal and health care services in a group setting that is residential in character and appearance in ways that optimize the physical and psychological independence of residents.'

Assisted living or close care is appropriate when older people begin to have difficulty keeping up with housekeeping chores, need help with dressing or bathing, or need reminders to take medicine. Yet they wish to remain independent and can easily do so if occasional help is available.

Who is assisted living and close care aimed at? The target population for residential forms of assisted living/close care is as follows:

- frail
- disabled
- confused
- incontinent but medically stable.

In essence the resident is a customer, with the provider being a broker or an arranger of care services. Assisted living and close care may therefore be described as housing with supportive services within a non-medical environment.

The nursing home traditionally provides more intensive care or nursing services with all services provided as a package. Yet many elderly people do not need nursing care. They simply need help with everyday activities. Studies such as that by Hamilton and Yatabes (1991) have indicated that an older person who is enabled to continue to live independently can remain healthier longer.

Nursing may be required by a person as they age but the incidence of the requirements for ongoing 24-hour licensed care tends only to be required by approximately 50 per cent of the existing United States nursing home residents. The figures are similar for the United Kingdom. In short the nursing home is an all-or-nothing form of care service. Assisted or close care housing offers a more flexible and affordable model of long-term care. At least 80 per cent of assisted living residents can look forward to remaining in their new homes without the need to transfer on a permanent basis to a nursing home.

Typical services may include:

- housekeeping
- daily bed making

- light housekeeping
- linen service
- assistance with bathing and dressing as needed
- breakfast, lunch and dinner served each day
- medication reminders
- monthly check of pulse rate, blood pressure and weight
- scheduled transportation
- 24-hour staff and emergency assistance
- licensed nurse available 7 days a week
- special dietary needs.

Alternative assisted living environments

The terms 'assisted living', 'close care', 'personal care' and 'residential care' are often used to describe the variety of care environments and supportive programmes. There are three basic generic types of assisted living and close care environments.

- the nursing home model
- the hotel model
- the residential model.

The nursing home model of assisted living is almost indistinguishable from a nursing home in terms of layout and amenities. Essentially it is a programme which is referred to as assisted living even though it is conducted within a nursing home environment.

The hotel model again resembles the nursing home layout, with the exception that the interiors are substantially upgraded, and may include carpets and improved lighting. In essence, this resembles a hotel with double loaded corridors and the residents' rooms being similar to a hotel room, i.e. single rooms with a single bed with bath but no pantry or kitchen area.

Because it is often difficult to distinguish both the nursing home and hotel models from that of a traditional nursing home, marketing of such units has proved to be difficult.

The residential model is based upon apartment-type units within an essentially residential setting. This resembles an apartment building with all areas designed for full wheelchair access. The programmes and activity spaces are designed for a frail elderly resident population. This model of residential long-term care first evolved in the Nether-

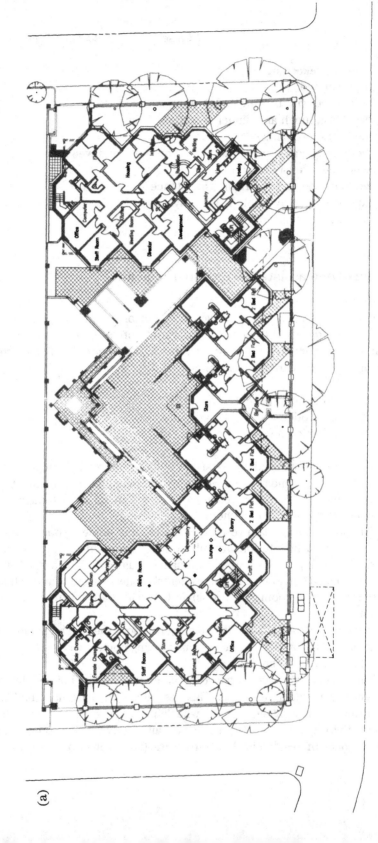

(a)

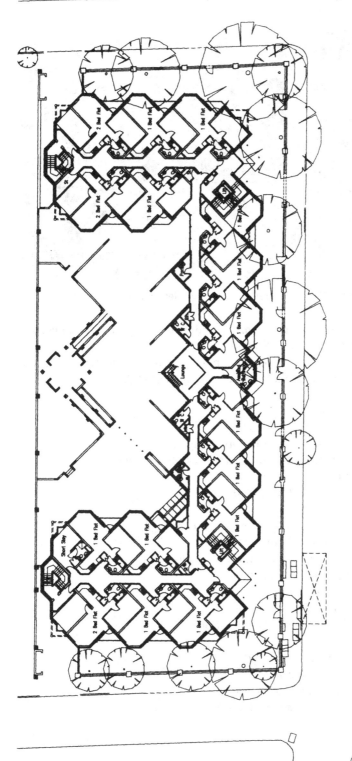

Fig. 9.1 Close care development, London; 37 self-contained apartments for older people, with care facilities provided on site. Client: Hornsey Housing Trust; architect: Salmon Speed. (a) ground floor plan, (b) first floor plan.

(b)

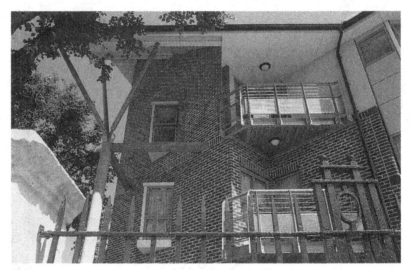

Fig. 9.2   Detail of balconies from close care development (Fig. 9.1).

lands and Scandinavia. It has since been adapted and developed extensively in the United States.

The differences between the medical and residential models of assisted living environments may be summarised thus

- Medical model
  - healthcare-type environment
  - similar to skilled care facility in layout and decor
  - minimal therapeutic effect from the environment
  - limited resident choices
  - perceived as part of skilled care
- Residential model
  - physically separated from skilled care facility
  - residential architectural character
  - residential type decor and furnishings
  - residential scale and layout
  - privacy – independence – dignity
  - choice of programme
- Assisted living design considerations
  - affordability
  - value for money invested
  - integration of services
  - residential scale and character
  - privacy as well as social interaction

- choice – control – autonomy
- orientation and wayfinding
- safety and security
- accessibility and functioning
- stimulation and challenge
- therapeutic environment
- familiarity
- aesthetics and appearance
- personalization
- adaptability.

Key programme and design issues

In reviewing future programmes each provider will have their own unique set of needs and requirements in the provision of appropriate environments for close care or city living stock. Yet there will be common threads running through each set of criteria in order to achieve best practice.

Based upon the same theme as first proposed by Cohen and Weisman (1991) in their research with Alzheimer's residents, the following is a summary of the twelve key design environmental issues to be addressed in the programming and design of close care and assisted living facilities. Apart from research undertaken at Reese, Lower, Patrick and Scott (Architects) and the published information, we would also particularly wish to acknowledge Victor Regnier's publication *Assisted Living, Housing For the Elderly* (1994) in the compiling of these design issues.

Affordability

The primary goal will be to create a caring, sensitive and attractive building which can fulfil a multitude of roles. Yet the building must also be functional and affordable, not only to achieve the intended construction budget, but also in terms of ongoing revenue and staffing costs. This requires a flow of creative ideas and a solid and dependable technical skills and construction cost management, as assisted living buildings will be of little use to anyone if no-one can afford to live there.

Safety and security

The building must provide a safe and secure environment for all users (residents, staff and visitors). Trip hazards and sharp or inappropriate rough finishes must all be avoided; security from dangerous equipment, and all relevant fire and safety regulations must all be borne in mind.

Environmental considerations

The residents must be able to see clearly and to distinguish objects, services, signs, clocks and changes of level. A combination of general and localized task lighting enables such features to be clearly defined. It is not only a matter of intensity of light provided but rather its ability to emphasize contrast.

The major interference with elderly people's speech comprehension tends to be difficulty in deciphering what has been said from the background level of sound. An acoustic environment should therefore be provided which reduces the background level of noise, particularly as discussed below.

Issues such as humidity, temperature control and air movement must be addressed to provide an environment tailored specifically to the special needs of an ageing occupant. The noise associated with climate control and air movement must be minimized so as not to interfere with the hearing ability of the residents.

With the foundation of a safe and secure environment for residents to live and for staff to work we can overlay the more complex design issues.

Privacy, independence, choice of control

The design should aim to incorporate the opportunity for residents to choose to do things for themselves. This might include the preparation of meals, washing and even some household chores; however, the choice to enjoy solitude and reflection should be respected both in the programme and in the design.

Ageing in place and the Peter Pan syndrome

Housing for the elderly has in many ways been overcrowded with retirement facilities that have assumed the Peter Pan syndrome – that once inside people will never age: many schemes have failed to allow or recognize the inevitability of ageing, which is an inherent demand placed not only on the building design but also upon the care service demands of the management organization. The key objective of close care or assisted living design is the ability to provide creative and appropriate solutions that will be able to flex and adapt to the changing needs of residents as they age in place. The design should aim to facilitate varying levels of care and support tailored to individual needs to be simply introduced into a resident's home as and when required. This will support the resident's desire to remain in their own home without the move to a nursing home for as long as possible.

Residential design and character

Close care and assisted living are residential models of long-term care. The building must express a residential quality physically, metaphorically and emotionally both in its architectural character and interior design.

Neighbourhood clusters

In terms of scale the design should be broken down into smaller groups and neighbourhoods. This is sometimes referred to as 'cluster design' or 'family groups'. This can vary from between eight and twelve assisted living apartments clustered within each family setting. The family groups can then take on a more residential scale, each becoming semi-autonomous from the rest of the facilities. Each family group can be designed to take on its own identity, thus helping to reinforce the importance of individuality and variation within the facility.

Corridor design

As residents may become less able over time to leave the facility, especially during inclement or hot weather, so the importance of the corridor comes into sharper focus. The institutional double loaded corridor should be avoided; instead the corridor needs to be designed as a space which may be enjoyed in its own right with opportunities to introduce daylight to emphasize as far as possible the sense of time as well as place. The corridor can take on the image of the street containing a variety of light, texture and scale, and being the space where spontaneous and informal contact may take place between residents as neighbours.

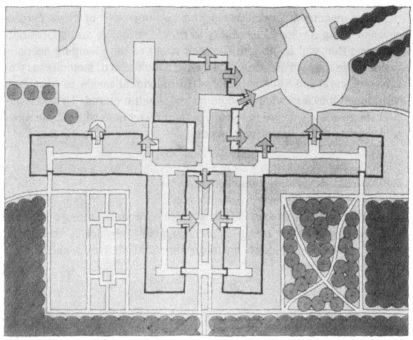

Fig. 9.3   Opportunities to connect a building's circulation areas to the outside can assist with orientation and help overcome the institutional effect of long and anonymous corridors. The above diagram illustrates a contemporary assisted living building in Greenville USA where at each opportunity the corridor offers the user a view out and an indication of the time of day or of the changing seasons and thereby utilizes nature as a natural orientation device.
Project: The Ridgewood St. Paul Homes, Greenville PA, USA. Architects: Reese Lower Patrick & Scott Ltd. Lancaster PA, USA.

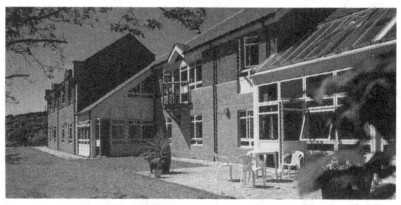

Fig. 9.4   Care housing expressed within a residential setting. Client: The Abbeyfield Gwent Extra Care Society Ltd; Architects: Salmon Speed Architects, London.

Conclusion

As assisted living and close care begin to replace the nursing home as a preferred model of long-term care so the healthcare services that are open to residents within the facility will also become the centres for home healthcare agencies. This could be combined with day care programmes. The key to the future of the provision of long-term care will be housing with services rather than the construction of special environments for the elderly. As assisted living continues to evolve, it is clear that there need to be a multitude of care models, designs and budgets. No one model could be advocated as a prototype. The 'one size fits all' approach advocated in some quarters demonstrates a basic misunderstanding of the real requirements of providing homes and services for the ageing. Provision of new assisted living and close care communities will provide an important bridge between the existing pattern of long-term care viewed within the medical framework and the future viewed within a flexible and adaptable residential community-based framework.

References

ALFAA (1990) *The Medicaid Home and Community Care Options Act.* Unpublished paper.

Benjamin, A. and Newcomer, R. (1986) *Board and care housing: an analysis of state differences.* Research on Aging **8:3**.

Blatter, A.Z. and Marty-Nelson, E. (1989) An Overview of the Low-Income Housing Tax Credit, in Mark S. Dennison (ed.) *Zoning and Planning Law Handbook.* Clark, Boardman Company Limited.

Calkins, M. (1988) *Designing for dementia: Planning Environments for the Elderly and Confused.* National Health Publishing, Owings Mills.

Cohen, U., Weisman, G., Ray, K. *et al.* (1988) *Environments for People with Dementia: Design Guide.* Center for Architecture and Urban Planning Research, University of Wisconsin-Milwaukee, Milwaukee.

Cohen, U. and Weisman, J. (1991). *Holding on to Home: Designing Environments for People with Dementia.* Johns Hopkins University Press, Baltimore.

Connerly, E. (1990) Housing trust funds: new resources for low-income housing. *Journal of Housing*, **47:2**.

Council of State Housing Agencies & National Association of State Units on Aging (1987) *Effects of the 1986 Tax Act on Financing of Housing for the Elderly.* Council of State Housing Agencies and NASUA, Washington DC.

Dobkin, L. (1989) *The Board and Care System: A Regulatory Jungle.* Consumer Affairs Program, Washington DC.

Guggenheim, J. (1988) Using tax credits: financing rehabilitation. *Journal of Housing* **45:4**.

Guggenham, J. (1988) Alternate Financing. *Journal of Housing* **45:4**.

Green, L. (1990) Humor and Lighthearted Activities, in Coons D. (ed). *Specialized Dementia Care Units*. The John Hopkins University Press, Baltimore.

Hamilton, R.V. and Yatabes, J. (1991) *Best Practices in Assisted Living*. National Eldercare Institute of Housing, University of Southern California.

Heumann, L. and Boldy, D. (1982). *Housing for the Elderly: Policy Formulation in Europe and North America*. St Martins Press, London.

Hoglund, D. (1985) *Housing for the Elderly: Privacy and Independence in Environments for the Aging*. Van Nostrand Reinhold, New York.

Kalymun, M. (1990) Toward a Definition of Assisted-Living, in Pastalan, L. (ed). *Optimizing Housing for the Elderly: Homes Not Houses*. The Hayworth Press, Inc., New York.

Jarvis, J. (1989) Seniors counsel wayward teens. *Senior World of Orange County.* **5:11**.

Kane, R., Illuston, L., Kane, R. and Nyman, J. (1990). *Meshing Services with Housing: Lessons from Adult Foster Care and Assisted Living in Oregon.* University of Minnesota, Long Term Care DECISIONS Resource Center, Minneapolis.

Laventhol and Horwath (1989) *Retirement Housing Industry 1988*. Laventhol & Horwath, Philadelphia.

Long Term Care National Resource Center at UCLA/USC (1989) *Assisted Living Resource Guide*. The Long Term Care National Resource Center at UCLA/USC, Los Angeles.

Mullen, A.J. (1989) *Nationwide Absorption Rates: The Critical Element in the Feasibility of Senior Living Projects*. Unpublished paper.

Mullen, A.J. (1991) The assisted living industry: an assessment. *Retirement Housing Report*, **Jan.**

National Association of Home Builders (1987) *Senior Housing. A Development and Management Handbook*. National Association of Home Builders of the United States, Washington DC.

Nenno, M.K. and Colyer, G.S. (1989) Trust funds: new trends in housing and finance. *Journal of Housing*, **446:1**.

Pynoos, J. (1990) Public policy and aging in place – identifying the problems and potential solutions, in David Tilson (ed.). *Aging in Place: Supporting the Frail Elderly in Residential Environment*. Scott, Foreman and Company, Illinois.

Regnier, V., Hamilton, H. and Yatabe, S. (1991) *Best Practices in Assisted Living*. National Eldercare Institute on Housing and Supportive Services, California.

Regnier, V. and Pynoos, J. (forthcoming). 'The Role of Environmental Design as a Therapeutic Intervention', in Birren, J., Sloan, B. and Choen, G. (eds) *Handbook of Mental Health and Aging*, Second Edition. New York: Academic Press.

Regnier, V. (1993). *Assisted Living, Housing for the Elderly*. Van Nostrand Reinhold, New York.

Seip, D. (1989a). First national assisted living industry survey. *Contemporary Long Term Care* **(12)** 7.

Seip, D. (1989b). Free-standing assisted living trends. *Contemporary Long Term Care.* **(12)**, 12.

Seip, D. (1989c). Tallying the first national assisted living survey. *Contemporary Long Term Care.* **(12)** 10.

Seip, D. (1990) *The Survival Handbook for Developers of Assisted Living.* The Seip Group, Boca Raton..

Special Committee on Aging. (1989). *Aging America: Trends and Projections Series* 101 E. U.S. Government Printing Office, Washington DC.

Stegman, M.A. (1986). *Housing Finance & Public Policy.* Van Nostrand Reinhold, New York.

Stryk, R., Page, D., Newman, S. *et al.* (1989) *Providing Supportive Services to the Frail Elderly in Federally Assisted Housing.* The Urban Institute Press, Washington DC.

Tuccillo, J.A. and Godman, J.L. (1983). *Housing Finance: A Changing System in The Reagan Era.* The Urban Institute Press, Washington DC.

United Nations (1982) *Report on the World Health Organisation.* Paper presented at the World Assembly on Aging in Vienna, July 26– August 6.

Valins, M. (1993) Adapting the facility to a tumultuous future nursing home. *Long Term Management.* Nov./Dec. 1993, **42**, 9.

Valins, M. (1993) *Primary Health Care Centers.* John Wiley and Sons, New York.

Valins, M. (1992) Design and Planning Elderly Care Facilities – The American Experience. *Hospital Development,* **2**, 10.

Valins, M. (1988) *Housing for Elderly People.* Butterworth Architecture, London.

Voeks, S. and Drinka, P. (1990) Participants' perception of a work therapy program in a nursing home. *Activities, Adaptations and Aging* **14.3**.

Weal, F. and Weal, F. (1988) *Housing for the Elderly: Options and Design.* Nicholas Publishing, New York.

Welch, P., Parker, V. and Zeisel, J. (1984) *Independence Through Interdependence.* Department of Elder Affairs, Commonwealth of Massachusetts.

Wilner, M. (1988) *Refining the Assisted Living Model to Include Persons with Limited Incomes and Smaller Resident Populations.* Milestone Management, Portland.

Further Reading

Carella, J. (1995) *Unlimited Options for Aging: Common Sense Answers from Scandinavia.* Hollis Publishing Co, Hollis NH, USA.

Wilson, K.B. (1990) Assisted Living: The Merger of Housing and Long Term Care Services. *Long Term Care Advances* **1**, p208.

Chapter 10
Long-term Care – A Residential Environment that is Striving to be a Home

Benyamin Schwarz

Introduction

There is a growing recognition that the nursing home in its current form has reached a turning point. Healthcare projections for the ageing population, the fiscal crisis in the long-term care system and the notion that older people and their families do not like the present types of building have driven the present nursing home to the limit. Continued reliance on the nursing home as the primary option for the frail elderly is thus neither economically wise nor socially desirable. This chapter examines the future of nursing home design and technology as two integral elements which may revolutionize such settings in the future.

The alien medical model

The myths surrounding old age in America are an important backdrop for any treatment of the issues surrounding long-term care. All cultures maintain ideals of ageing and old age which reflect the paradoxes of later life: that ageing is a source of wisdom and suffering, of spiritual growth and physical decline, of honour and vulnerability.

Several cultures have believed that ageing should be accepted and that it should be in part a time of preparation for death. American society is different in this sense as Thomas Cole noted in *The Journey of Life* (1992). It often seems that Americans prefer to think of ageing as hardly more than another disease, to be fought and rejected:

> Since the early twentieth century and especially after World War II, public discussion of ageing has taken place largely within the framework of science and medicine. By medical and social means, scientists have effectively labelled ageing as a problem that we can solve (or at least manage) given enough basic research and intervention.

As a result of this notion the phenomenon and experience of ageing have been placed within the medical paradigm as an individual pathology to be treated and cured. Most Americans die of chronic and progressive illnesses such as heart disease, stroke and cancer. These age-related illnesses and disabilities are usually irremediable; cure is the exception not the rule. Therefore the current emphasis on physical and medical aspects of care and the application of medical ways of thinking in a nursing home environment seem paradoxical. There are of course some residents who can benefit from medical treatment and restorative therapy. However the nature of the majority of the serious disabilities that are associated with old age means that they are neither curable nor capable of rehabilitation. Nevertheless the medical model that migrated from the acute care of the hospital to the nursing home has misguided the environmental design of the setting for the past thirty years. As G.J. Agich (1993) noted, despite the fact that its 'underlying values and beliefs are widely recognised as inappropriate'.

No typical nursing home exists. Indeed enormous diversity is present in most American nursing homes, as Vladeck (1980) noted in his now classic *Unloving Care*. Still, an ordinary nursing home looks, feels and even smells like a medical facility. Like general hospitals, nursing homes have long corridors loaded with rows of wide open doors to residents' rooms on both sides. A waist-high railing between the doors provides a support for residents who wander the corridors and manoeuvre past wheelchairs. The corridors are crowded with utility carts for clean and soiled laundry, medication carts and people strolling the halls or sitting in their chairs against the walls. The commonly used vinyl floors reflect the glare from stark fluorescent lighting. The walls are painted in institutional colours and display paintings of rural scenes and still life arrangements. Odours of urine, disinfectant, medications and laundry permeate the air. Residents' television sets are constantly on and the murmur of the game show whistles and applause, commercial jingles and soap opera dialogue serve as a cacophonous 'muzak' backdrop to nursing home life, interrupted periodically by the public address system which frequently echoes through the corridors. Figure 10.1 gives some idea of these surroundings.

Typically, cramped in the middle of each unit is a nursing station. The high-fronted desk which enables staff to look out into corridors is covered with books and manuals, racks of residents' charts and miscellaneous supplies. Staff members sit behind the desk and talk to residents in front of them, write charts or talk on the telephone. They maintain records and distribute medications even though most care focuses on occupational and physiotherapy and is provided by aides

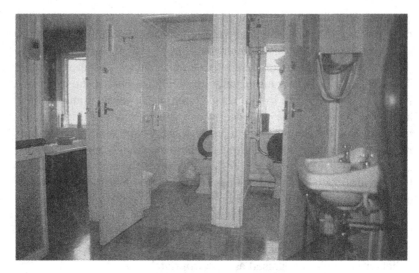

Fig. 10.1   Communal toileting area in a nursing unit.

rather than by trained nurses. Each unit has a room where residents are bathed in cubicles separated by curtains. This procedure is directed more to staff convenience than residents' privacy and dignity. One dining room is located on every floor and it is also used for other recreational purposes. Inside the room there are several institutional tables and chairs and a television set. The floor is tiled for easy maintenance and the walls are painted in hospital-like colours.

Residents' rooms are stark, most have two single beds and one window. In such rooms one resident will be nearer the window than the other who will be in the darker side of the room nearer the bathroom. A sliding privacy curtain separates the beds. Each resident has an emergency call button, one night table, one small chair and limited cupboard space. Residents share a lavatory, a sink and a mirror. The rooms are just large enough to accommodate the furniture. The administration of many nursing homes encourages residents to bring memorabilia from home, yet the shortage of wall and surface space effectively limits residents from making the rooms reflect their lives, families or interests.

Despite the fact that most people who are admitted to nursing homes reside there permanently, little is done to satisfy their many non-medical needs. Nursing home systems, procedures and environments are not designed to make the residents' lives more natural or meaningful. The overriding theme of most literature on nursing homes reflects that many Americans view placement in a nursing home as joyless and terrible. As quoted by J.S. Savishinsky (1991):

'Such institutions are seen as the last resort of those who can no longer help themselves. In the apparent uselessness of one's later years they symbolise rejection and they sometimes rub the salt of neglect into the moral wounds of marginality. This sad spoilt image of late life contrasts with equal extreme myth of the golden age of old age, a once hallowed but now respected truth that people no longer believe in them. The imagination of our culture has transformed the old dream into a new nightmare.'

Nursing homes can be frightening and depressing places. They remind us of our own mortality and present a threat to our human sense of wellbeing. When we visit these institutions we are reminded of the inevitable time when most of us will face ultimate powerlessness and vulnerability. We fear that if we live long enough we too may one day meet our fate in a nursing home. The very existence of this setting threatens a sense of what normal life ought to be. We may even conclude that nursing homes ought not to exist.

At the same time nursing homes are still the primary shelters to which exhausted families turn when elderly dependents cannot manage in a home environment and when other options of long-term care are unavailable or ineffective.

Evolution of a misguided model

McClure (1968) attributed the growth of the nursing home in the care of the elderly to a consequence of three essential developments. First, there is an increasing proportion of older persons in the population. Second, as society became increasingly urbanized the character of domestic living structures changed with a nuclear family assuming much greater importance than the extended family. The modernization theory that originated at the same time warned about the potential in industrialized societies for the disintegration of the family and the abandonment of aged persons (Hashimoto, 1993). Third, the evolution of new social policies demanded a secure old age, and led to the passage of measures such as social security and later Medicaid.

The nursing home is a relatively new type of building. Its origin can be traced in the United States to the 1954 Hill-Burton Act which replaced federal legislation supporting hospital construction (Collopy *et al.*, 1991). In the United Kingdom nursing homes were incorporated into the National Health Service Act of 1946 and the establishment of the National Health Service in 1948. Prior to these enactments nursing homes were primarily residential facilities, custodial in character, which cared for residents with chronic illnesses and disabilities. Doctors' involvement in these facilities was very limited. The inclusion of the nursing home in the Hill-Burton Act and the UK National Health Service legislation transformed them by definition into medical facilities and led to the initial creation of standards for their physical construction and design. Nursing homes first emerged as alternative homes for the elderly who could not stay with their families, or those without family and for the poor.

Hickey (1981) noted that:

'Over time however, geographic separation and smaller homes have made the family context a less likely focus of care for those older people with adequate family support and financial resources. Given these developments it was not surprising that the nursing home emerged in the social institutional image of a hospital rather than an alternative home. As the key decision makers in the process, physicians find it simpler to transfer patients from one medical institution to another.'

The improvement of hospitals as curative remedial facilities called for a division of labour and efficiency in order to separate the historical sheltering function of the hospital from the provision of acute care (Thomas, 1969). Nursing homes were thus integrated into the prevailing hospital concept of 'progressive patient care', in which patients were moved from one level of care intensity to another as their condition changed; this of course emphasized time management and efficiency. An efficient nursing home unit in a hospital typically has had three care sections: high dependency, intermediate and self care. Nursing homes were expected to be at the final stage of institutionalization where chronically ill patients who have surpassed acute care levels can receive maximum care at a lower cost.

Principles of efficiency and time management have found their way into therapeutic environments from origins in the industrial assembly line where actions and space became defined units with labels such as events, tasks and activities. Time was considered controllable and not simply the result of external natural forces. Efficiency promised that adherence to a particular sequence of activities in a timely manner could produce certain outcomes. Moreover, within the scope of such predictability the relative merits of action, especially in terms of time and effort could be defined clearly and then compared, thus establishing the background for minimum standards and reimbursement systems.

Consequently two central forces have controlled the environmental design of present nursing homes in addition to the provision of care concerns:

- Governmental funding has flowed to nursing homes over the years, carrying with it the priorities and reflections of the fiscal acute care system.
- Strict regulations have been developed within a tradition that emphasized satisfaction of medical and custodial needs rather than residents' quality of life. This is evident in the total environment of the nursing home which isolates and thereby controls the daily lives of residents.

Agich (1993) states:

'Since staff are primarily oriented towards pursuing medically related activities, the dominant mode of discourse the schedule and work evaluations, are based on the performance of such specific tasks as bathing, feeding or toilet assistance – the full effects of this orientation for the autonomy of elders go unnoticed. The medically defined objectives rarely take into account the elder as an experiencing subject and person who is the object of care.'

Furthermore, the care given to residents in nursing homes simply does not realize therapeutic goals. The underlying problem is not the issue of custodial care and the inability to restore health or wellbeing but 'unclarity or controversy regarding the basic meaning of health or wellbeing for an institutionalised frail elderly' (Agich, 1993).

The ideological contradiction that seems to impede the nursing home from fulfilling its potential as a resident-focused care facility may be attributed to the fact that western society is increasingly driven by two opposing demands – a cultural drive for maximum autonomy on the one hand and an economic drive for efficiency on the other.

Bell (1973) argues that the economy and the culture of the post-industrial society pull in diametrically opposed directions; the economy demands increased specialization and limits whereas the culture promises augmentation of the self. This contradiction is expressed in governmental payment systems and regulations of nursing homes and in day-to-day operations of nursing homes. The mainstream liberal ideology of the 'ageing enterprise' holds that research practice and policy all work together to benefit the elderly (Estes, 1979). Researchers in the field of the environment in ageing have subscribed to this view and designers also have given credence to the architectural premise that knowledge of basic principles of human behaviour leads to better environments. Celebrating in what Robert Butler phrased as the 'Union of Science and Advocacy' (Butler, 1975), designers of nursing homes have followed two theoretical design modes during the past decades: the prosthetic mode and the therapeutic mode.

The prosthetic mode

Implicit in the provision of facilities for the elderly has been the assumption that both physical and interpersonal aspects of the environment affect outcome. Consequently early studies of environment and ageing tend to emphasize the role of the physical environment as a demand on human competence. Several theoretical models have focused on the prosthetic role of the environment. Briefly stated, they suggest that human ability to function is a result of interaction between individual capabilities and environmental support. Matches of individual competence with the environment of a particular structure happen within a zone or range of adaptability. Mismatches that create over-support lead to dependency, whereas those that create under-support can result in diminished levels of functioning and increased levels of stress. This prosthetic mode developed within an intellectual tradition which believed that humans are adaptive organisms which react predictably to given stimuli. Existing literature from this viewpoint has emphasized space over place. It has focused on the fact that ageing and particularly extreme old age, bring physical and sensual limitations which alter an individual's ability to negotiate the environment.

As a result nursing home design has stressed the provision of appropriate space and the functional aspects of the environment. However designers have disregarded the inherent meaning of place for residents, staff and visitors, and have made an effort to transform it into an appealing environment.

The therapeutic mode

This school of thought emphasizes that both empirical and theoretical support exist for the therapeutic role of the physical setting in the care of frail elderly people. Interest in the therapeutic potential of the environment has grown during the past two decades. Consequently there have been numerous attempts in recent years to develop guidelines for design facilities that can contribute to therapeutic care for frail elderly people. The most obvious example is special care dementia units designed and marketed as settings which can slow, or in some cases reverse, the declines expected over time in the behaviour of people with dementia.

The therapeutic model is nothing new. Early expression of the therapeutic mode is explicit in another architectural precedent. At the zenith of their confidence in the 1920s, modern architects emotionally proclaimed the beginning of an exhilarating new era. Illness and inhibition, social strife and obfuscation would end, and in their place would rise a new spirit of vigorous good health, order and rationality. The key aspect of the modern architect's position was a deep confidence in the efficacy of the new rigorous and even scientific rationality they proposed to apply to design. Pervasive physical presence of light, sun and fresh air was sought in building design and in theory manifestation, not only because the modern architects were so confident that the new promoted good health but also because they were such potent symbols of the new world which modern architecture promised to bring into being. The tuberculosis sanatorium eventually became the single most convincing public symbol of the new architecture because the actual medical treatment then recommended for tuberculosis (lots of light, sun and fresh air) coincided so exactly with the cultural metaphor of good health central to the philosophy of modern architecture. Central to this concept was the notion that some match exists between the physical form and content of the setting and the programmes, policies and organizational structure of a care facility. Unfortunately the functionalization of nursing home architecture and the transformation of care into a set of operational rules appear to contradict the therapeutic role of this environment. Nursing home design seemed to intensify rather than emulate the violation of personal privacy and resident autonomy resulting from physical impairment.

The therapeutic mode emphasizes the interaction of architectural, organizational and social factors in an effort to break away from the institutional model of the nursing home. The recurrent theme in this mode is an attempt to make institutions more domestic or homelike.

Whilst elements of both the prosthetic mode and the therapeutic mode will very likely influence future nursing home design, the crucial cultural change towards such design will arise from two elements:

- provision of care rather than cure for our elders
- the growing awareness of a person's experience of physical space as a personally meaningful place.

Futurecare: reconstructing the nursing home

Whilst prognostication by designers often stems from plain curiosity it also arises from their wish to ensure that current plans will not become obsolete or redundant in the future. Design and technology will reshape the long-term care landscape and may even force the nursing home building type to disappear and to be replaced by more residential environments. However progress will not be a panacea.

By the year 2030 the nursing home population is expected to reach 5.3 million in the United States, another 13.8 million elderly in the community will need help with the activities of daily living (US Bi Partisan Commission on Comprehensive Health Care (1990)). These predictions may however be modified as a vast technology has become prominent. Visionary experts predict that over the next 20 years society will experience an explosion in healthcare technology. Much of that scientific advancement is expected to come from the field of biotechnology. According to optimistic predictions the understanding of biological processes and the cause of disease will lead to new treatments and new cures for heart disease, cancer and AIDS. A major effort will focus on the prevention of diseases associated with ageing such as Alzheimer's disease, diabetes and osteoporosis.

Callahan (1987) argues that as a society we need to set limits to healthcare for the elderly. He argues that we have the ability to extend life, and since the elderly neither have a reasonable chance for productive life and nor does society as a whole have (or wish to allocate) infinite resources necessary for intensive medical care for the elderly, an age-based rationing of medical care is the fairest way to allocate these resources. He claims that

'the future goal of medical science should be to improve the quality of old people's lives, not lengthen them. In this long standing ambition to forestall death, medicine has reached its last frontier in the care of the aged.'

Other than economical and social implications the rationale for this approach stems from the fact that 'there is no perfect correlation between health and happiness, between length of life and satisfaction with life, or between the health of individuals and their common good as a community'.

Whilst the ramifications of these questions are not clear, the expansion of other technologies may alter the boundaries and limitations surrounding the settings where care is provided. Sophisticated technology based on miniaturization may transport part of high-tech care into individual homes and the development of the neighbouring environments will encourage more independent living. Communication options and control devices will provide more connections to the immediate environment and beyond. Devices such as walk-in bath tubs, adjustable height showers with comfortable seats and arm rests, adjustable height sinks, water closets, and other kinds of equipment will increase the level of resident independence and will assist staff in providing care. Advances in transportation, prosthetic devices and kitchen appliances will aid those individuals requiring such assistance. Finally the use of robotics as assisted tools for living will become more common. There is no question that applications of innovative technology will be part of long-term care service delivery. Rather than trying to predict the future, however, we need to dream it up.

The futuristic model

The invention of the future type of nursing home has to be based on a premise that no amount of buyer medical research and technological intervention can bring ageing fully under the control of the human will or desire. The myth of cure is costly in human and financial terms. Compassion is the best medicine and that is the reason that the future nursing home should focus on care and on meeting imaginable and realizable goals. Technology and environmental design in long-term care settings should aspire to meet the following three goals.

- *Provide conditions to meet bodily needs:* The role of technology in meeting this goal would be one of enabling every individual to live full biographical (not necessarily biological) life span. Efforts to reduce morbidity as well as efforts to diminish causes of premature death would be a primary objective of this aspiration.
- *Maximize attributes to meet cognitive and emotional needs:* Environmental design and technology should support programmes and policies which assist people in achieving a stable mental and emotional state. Sensory and social stimulation should be adjusted to maintain balance. The environment should encourage socialization, support autonomy and control and protect the need for privacy.
- *Support opportunities to meet functional needs:* Environmental design should afford engagement in meaningful activities, rehabilitation and other therapies that help to maintain adequate functional capacities and self esteem.

These aspirations and ideals are goals towards which we might strive. Nevertheless we have to be able to accept the limits of human lives and the tensions between our aspirations and our social economic realities. Designers have other significant roles.

Restructuring nursing homes – sense of place

Where a person is assigned meaning both in and by a place, time and space assume particular unique values in this context. Von Meiss (1986) states that: 'they cease to be mathematical abstraction or a subject of aesthetics; they acquire an identity and become a reference for our existence'.

The present nursing home is loaded with hostile meanings. It is charged with identifiable values that are apparent to residents and to others. These values suggest modes of behaviour. The nursing building type is associated with events which it accommodates, with frailty, with other similar places and with frightening events. Designers of this setting must therefore refer especially to the idea of place and not only to utilitarian aspects, aesthetic principles or constructional rules. In other words they have to be able to unite these elements in order to sustain the idea of place.

Conclusion

Environmental designers cannot dictate the value of places. However they can, by reference based on observation, reflection and research, provide a framework which may accommodate those particular situations which are common to all humans. The sense of place associated with nursing homes can be reconstructed to offer greater potential for meeting people, for being happy, for participating in healthy and familiar activities, for stimulating associations of ideas and memories and even for dreaming. The future nursing home environment should apply design and technology to support residents, staff and families in a fashion that is not cohesive and that creates appealing meaningful place.

References

Agich, G.J. (1993). *Autonomy and Long-Term Care*. Oxford University Press, New York.

Bell, D. (1973). *The Coming of Post-Industrial Society*. Basic Books, New York.

de Beauvoir, S. (1972) *The Coming of Age*. Putman, New York.

Butler, R.N. (1975) *Why survive: Being Old in America*. Harper and Row, New York.

Callahan, D. (1987). *Setting Limits: Medical Goals in an Aging Society*. Simon & Schuster Inc., New York.

Callahan, D. (1990) *What Kind of Life. The Limits of Medical Progress*. Simon & Schuster Inc., New York.

Callahan, D. (1991) Limiting health care for the old. In N.S. Jecker (Ed). *Aging and Ethics: Philosophical Problems in Gerontology*. Humana Press, New Jersey.

Cohen, U. and Weisman, G.D. (1991) *Holding On To Home: Designing Environments for People with Dementia*. The Johns Hopkins University Press, Baltimore.

Cole, T. (1992) *The Journey of Life. A Cultural History of Aging in America*. Cambridge University Press, Cambridge.

Collopy, B., Boyle, B. and Jennings, B. (1991). *New Directors in Nursing Home Ethics*. A Hastings Center Report. Special Supplement, March–April 1991.

Coons, D. (1985) Alive and well at Wesley Hall. *A Journal of Long Term Care*, **21** (2).

Estes, C. (1979) *The Aging Enterprise*. Jossey-Bass, San Francisco.

Hashimoto, A. (1993) Family relations in later life: a cross-cultural perspective. *Generations*, **XVII**, 4.

Hickey, T. (1981). *Long-term Care of the Elderly: Consumer Issues and Perspectives*. Gerontological Research Institute, Washington.

McClure, E. (1968) *More than a Roof*. Minnesota Historical Society, St Paul, Minn.

Moody, H.R. (1988) *Abundance of Life. Human Development Policies for an Ageing Society*. Columbia University Press, New York.

Moody, H.R. (1992) *Ethics in an Ageing Society*. The Johns Hopkins University Press, Baltimore.

Rubinstein, R.L. and Parrell, P.A. (1992) Attachment to Place and the Representation of the Life Course by the Elderly. In *Place Attachment* (eds I. Altuain & S. Low). Plenum Press, New York.

Savashinsky, J.S. (1991) *The Ends of Time; Life and Work in a Nursing Home*. Bergin & Garvely, New York.

Schwartz, B. (1992) *Designing Public Places for Private Lives; A Study of the Design Process of Long Term Care Settings*. Doctorial Thesis, University of Michigan.

Thomas, W.C. (1969) *Nursing Homes and Public Policy: Drift and Decision in New York State*. Cornell University Press, Ithaca, NY.

US Bi Partisan Commission on Comprehensive Health Care (19990). *A Call for Action: The Pepper Commission Final Report*. US Government Printing Office, Washington.

Vladek, B.C. (1980) *Unloving Care: The Nursing Home Tragedy*. Basic Books, New York.

Von Meiss, P. (1988) *Elements of Architecture from Form to Place*. Chapman & Hall, London.

Chapter 11
Nursing Home 2000

Martin S. Valins

Introduction

Despite all the care, love and devotion of the staff of nursing homes, most are faced with a daily battle against a built environment that typically just does not work. Both the United Kingdom and the United States are littered with examples of nursing homes that cut against the grain of what management and staff attempt to do in terms of their programmes of care and support for the people they serve.

Is the problem just bad design? Do architects fail to create the right solutions? No. The problem of nursing home design goes far deeper. It is a fundamental issue that the concept of the licensed or registered nursing home has become out of sync with the needs and expectations of our elderly population who require long-term care.

The root cause of the problem of the nursing home environments is that they were originally conceived out of a hospital model, an environment best suited to short-term medical treatment. It is only recently that we have begun to distinguish old age from illness. Becoming old does not necessarily imply that one will become ill or need constant medical supervision.

Yet when licensing legislation was first drafted in the 1960s, both in the United States and the United Kingdom, it automatically assumed that long-term care would take place in an environment best suited to the treatment of illness rather than the promotion of wellness and the right of the individual to privacy, dignity and independence.

The nursing home environment today is driven by a plethora of codes and regulations written in a language of the past. Most nursing home administrators consider the regulations a hinderance to the type of environments and care programmes they would prefer to see. The codes and regulations rightly protect and enforce certain life safety issues, but beyond that there is little mention in the codes of the quality of life that a resident can expect from within a code dominated environment. With this in mind it is now high time for the codes and regulations in their present form to go. They are no longer relevant to our long-term needs, and there would be few who would mourn their passing.

The future

To create a vision for the future, that is, how nursing homes could look in the next decade, it is important that we return to basics. Let us for a moment sweep away the regulations, the reimbursement procedures, even the words nursing home, and imagine what type of environment we would create that would best serve human beings needing support during their final years of life. It would perhaps be a place of contemplation and companionship, a place of light and warmth, a place of love and hope, a place of peace and yet also of activities, of music, of memories, of laughter. It would also be a place to cry, to be alone, and to do as one chooses.

What a contrast these simple yet fundamental human requirements seem from the typical reality of the nursing home environment with its double loaded corridors, shared bedrooms, fluorescent strip lighting and unsightly nursing stations. The nursing home of the future will be radically different from our current model. Indeed the question is no longer if the nursing home should change but rather how quickly it can change to keep pace with the changing market.

Some would argue that an ageing population will secure an increasing demand for nursing beds well into the next century. However, available research suggests that the age wave may indeed beach the nursing home in its current state while the market moves upshore.

In terms of consumer demand and new models of care, plus the revised financial reimbursement packages envisaged on both sides of the Atlantic, the nursing home must stand as the most vulnerable component of long-term care. As with any evolutionary cycle, the key to survival will be to adapt or die. That is the challenge each nursing home provider faces in taking an outmoded building type into the next century.

The writing is already on the wall. In June 1995 the US Census Bureau showed a slower than expected increase in the nation's nursing home population during the 1980s, providing evidence that growing old need not inevitably lead to a life in a nursing home.

Researchers have indicated that these numbers bear out other studies in the United States and elsewhere in northern Europe, that fewer elderly people are suffering from the kinds of disabilities which have historically confined them to nursing homes. This improvement also stems from healthier lifestyles and medical technological advances that aid recovery from strokes, broken hips and the traumas of ageing. More importantly during the last decade, there has been an expansion of services which allow the elderly to stay out of nursing homes including the advent and growth of community healthcare and assisted living or close care forms of housing. These options have been eagerly welcomed by an elderly population who consistently say in consumer surveys that they dread the thought of having to live out their last years in a nursing home.

Options for improvement

So how can nursing home boards prepare for the inevitability of future change? Despite the many negative aspects of existing nursing home environments, there are in fact many opportunities which are waiting to be explored. Essentially there are four options which need to be considered:

- do nothing
- convert to close care/assisted living
- integrate as a community care resource
- implement programmes for sub-acute/patient hotel programmes.

Appraising the options

In any option appraisal it is sometimes helpful to prepare a checklist of the criteria that those options will be appraised against. Below are just some of the key issues that could form a checklist.

- What are the current occupancy levels at the home? Has there been a shift in demand? If so where?
- How many residents actually require 24-hour nursing care as opposed to more personal care programmes?
- How well located is the nursing home in comparison with other community care services?
- What percentage of the residents are private payers and what has been the trend over the last 10 years?
- What is the physical condition of the home – will it require upgrading in any case simply to improve the existing nursing home programmes?

- Is the building capable of being adapted structurally?
- Is there land to expand upon?
- What will be the impact of health care reform on the facilities?
- What is the local competition doing?
- What relationship does the home have with local hospitals?

It is also helpful when appraising options to look at the bigger picture, and to consider long-term planning. It would also be helpful at this stage for the provider of the nursing home to review its original mission for the home and to decide whether healthcare reform on both sides of the Atlantic will almost certainly imply moving the focus of healthcare delivery away from hospitals and towards community-based satellite healthcare facilities. Those nursing homes already located close to their local communities will be well positioned to take on and develop this role. The nursing home as a healthcare resource centre would therefore offer a variety of health and care programmes. Of course, there will still be a need for skilled residential care but this option would at least offer nursing homes the opportunity to diversify their services.

Forward-thinking providers and architects are building flexibility into plans for nursing homes. Figures 11.1 and 11.2 illustrate how resident rooms in a nursing home have been designed to facilitate the option to convert to an assisted living programme.

Programmes for sub-acute care and patient care hotels

Sub-acute care is perhaps going back full circle to where the nursing home began within the medical arena. Patients whose medical condition still requires 24-hour monitoring and perhaps some medical intervention, but are no longer in a critical condition are generally referred to as sub-acute.

As hospitals become centres of high-tech, short term, acute intervention, so there is a growing need for that longer second stage of recovery to take place out of the expensive environment of the hospital and closer within the fabric of the community. In northern Europe such programmes are referred to as 'Patient Hotels'. These are less expensive environments in which to accommodate patients more in a hotel type rather than acute medical environment. (A more detailed account of sub-acute care is offered in Chapter 16).

Sub-acute care is increasingly gaining recognition as an important level of care offering focused patient care and cost savings. Sub-acute care is typically 25–50% less expensive than a similar acute care setting.

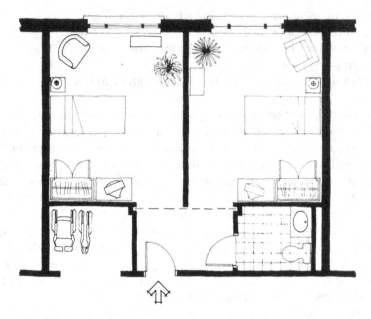

Fig. 11.1   Resident room layout for nursing care.

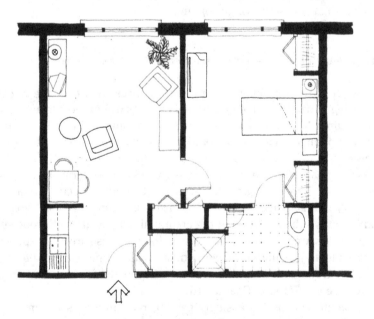

Fig. 11.2   Option for low-cost conversion to assisted living.
(Copyright figs 11.1 and 11.2, RLPS Architects, Lancaster Pa., USA.)

The length of stay in a sub-acute centre averages between two weeks to six months. Many medically complex patients face extensive periods of recovery. As a result of the increased reimbursement rate potential, the sub-acute market may well become cluttered. As opposed to converting to assisted living the typical nursing home layout would be more compatible with the space requirements for sub-acute programmes. Engineering services would need to be upgraded but this could generally be accommodated within the existing building shell with perhaps a few alterations and additions.

However, if a nursing home were to develop its interest in the sub-acute care market, it would need to consider the implication of introducing a somewhat different medical culture into its care programs.

In addition a home would need to be aware of, and if necessary, revisit its mission in relation to the following:

- Sub-acute care is focused upon recuperation and is driven by the need to achieve a higher through-put of patients. It is short term, *not* long term care. Patients' expectations are to be treated and to recover.
- Sub-acute care relies upon the ability to attract patients from alliances with health care organizations. If a home wished to pursue the sub-acute care market, it would need to align itself with block purchasing organizations such as hospitals, and managed care groups.
- Sub-acute care is not necessarily an age related problem – so this could entail serving younger adults.
- Sub-acute care will be a managed program involving cost effectiveness and turn-over efficiency.

In conclusion, no doubt further options and opportunities may be on the horizon for the nursing home. One thing is certain, the days of the nursing home as a preferred model for long-term care are numbered. The future change is inevitable and nursing home administrators and provider organizations should begin now to plan and chart their course strategically for the future.

Chapter 12
Dementia Care

Martin S. Valins

Introduction

The increase in the number of reported cases of Alzheimer's disease may be directly related to the increasing number of people surviving beyond the ago of 80, where the incidence of this chronic condition can affect one in five. Alzheimer's disease was probably always with us but has now come into sharper focus in tandem with our ageing population. Alzheimer's disease is a progressive, irreversible disease, characterized by degeneration of the brain cells and commonly leading to severe dementia. It is named after the German physician who first described it, Dr Alois Alzheimer (1864–1915).

While the condition will probably remain incurable well into the 21st century, there is a growing body of opinion and some research to suggest that the environment can play a therapeutic role in supporting care programmes to stabilize and alleviate some, although not all, of the symptoms of dementia. These are as follows:

- loss of memory and the ability to think clearly
- loss of ability to make judgements
- loss of inhibitions, e.g., performing private functions in public
- loss of emotional function and control (people who have been caring, loving people become greedy, selfish and aggressive)
- loss of ability to make 'if–then' connections, e.g., *if* I drop a lighted cigarette on the carpet *then* that could start a fire
- wandering (which can be a combination of loss of memory and a subconscious urge to escape from an intolerable situation).

The link between providing a better quality of life and the role of the environment specifically relating to the care of the people with dementia has been discussed in three publications: *Nursing Home Renovation: Design for Reform* by Dr Lorraine G. Hyatt, *Holding on to Home* by Dr

Gerald Weisman and Dr Uriel Cohen and *Designing for Dementia* by Dr Margaret Calkins.

The research and information contained in the above works has a direct relevance not only for environments which we should consider today and more importantly it offers clear directions as to how best we should shape future care environments for people with dementia and cognitive impairment.

Five myths about dementia

Hyatt (1991) describes five myths relating to the nursing home. This method of addressing myths has been adapted specifically for people with dementia.

The first myth identified by Dr Hyatt is that all people with dementia are the same. Although the majority of sufferers will be aged 80+ the condition nevertheless appears to affect a diverse cross-section of cultures, class and background. In addition, dementia cannot be described as a constant condition. The degree to which the disease will affect an individual will vary from day to day, even minute to minute.

The second myth is that people with dementia require specially designed units. The majority of the nursing homes that exist today are really first generation arising from government support programmes and built on what we knew best, which was the medical model. If all nursing homes were to be redesigned away from a medical towards a residential model, and if they all contained the positive features of light, space and scale, as required for a special care unit, then the need for specially designed units would diminish. Even bearing this in mind, it is still the case that approximately 60 per cent of nursing home population will present symptoms of dementia.

That design of the unit comes before the design of the therapeutic programme constitutes the third myth. In dementia care we need to focus more on personal space not just the whole – what one touches, hears, sees and smells. The preparation of a thorough programme is therefore fundamental. The building is at best a vehicle for a programme, and as soon as the design predetermines the programme, then various options are reduced. This is particularly important when one considers that the field of caring for people with dementia is still an evolving field. It is therefore important to remember that the design is a component part of the programme and not the other way round.

Dr Hyatt's fourth myth is that environmental design is related to problem solving and three dimensions. The information we gain from the environment is a complex combination which we receive and process through all our senses including:

- sight
- hearing
- smell
- taste
- touch.

Layered over this are our own unique cultural, social and economic values and expectations which help us to make value judgements as to whether we feel comfortable within any human space.

So when considering the most appropriate environment for a person with dementia it is not just a matter of square feet but a combination of light, touch, smell, sound and space, all interconnecting with our own individual patterns of expectations and value judgements.

Finally, it is believed in many quarters that there is one model of care in terms of design and layout that works. This is possibly harmful, as there are inherent dangers and limited value in simply looking at other special care units and evaluating how they look. Furthermore, because the success of any scheme will rely upon a multi-dimensional criteria of factors, the 'one size fits all' approach cannot be applied to the complexities of special care. Yet it can be argued that codes and regulations imply that there is just one preferred way.

Ten goals for the future

Cohen and Weisman (1991) have managed to encompass the complex issues of a relationship between the environment and therapeutic benefits by offering design-orientated goals. Based upon this theme we can consider 10 social and environmental goals which will need to be considered for any future care design programme for the care of people with dementia. There is consciously an overlap between these goals as in reality there should be seamless interplay between the criteria for each of the following.

Provide secure shelter, warmth and food

For people with dementia, a priority is to ensure safety, security and nourishment. Such patients represent a particularly vulnerable client group in terms of safety and security hazards due to both the onset of cognitive as well as physical impairment.

Support those abilities not totally impaired by dementia

Much of the literature apart from those books previously mentioned, has tended to concentrate on what a person cannot do instead of concentrating on what a person with dementia can do. It is therefore important that future facilities can support the normal activities of daily living and support a person's independence within their dependence.

Ensure an appropriate range of environmental and sensual stimulation and information

Stimulation is the arousal of our senses from the information we receive from the environment. Many existing nursing homes already promote over stimulation, usually of the wrong kind: noxious smells, the clanging of service trolleys, and footsteps thumping against hard surfaces. In addition, glare and inappropriate lighting all combine to provide irritants to a caring environment. On the other hand, environments that provide too little stimulation can be just as much of a hindrance to a therapeutic outcome. Instead there should be an objective of aiming for a variety of different levels of stimulation tailored to individual need so that an individual may choose where he or she will feel most comfortable. In particular, a view onto a quiet and tranquil courtyard can be contrasted with the participation or observation in cooking, eating and space to exercise. Stimulation of the senses is not just concerned with light and space, however. It is also related to sound (music), touch, smell and the feeling of a cool summer breeze on one's face.

Support and reinforce people to know where they are in time and space

Wayfinding is finding one's way from A to B – we can all suffer from the frustration of being lost in a confusing environment. Orientation is knowing where one is in time and space. Landmarks such as clocks or paintings will enable residents with dementia to read the environment to know where they are in both contexts. For residents who may have previously lived in a self-contained house, corridors will represent a new experience and therefore the design of the corridor will be particularly important. As residents may become building-bound so the corridor could take on the image of the street, thereby containing all the necessary variety of light, texture and scale. The use of daylight is also important within circulation spaces to emphasize as far as possible the sense of time as well as space. However, a frequent problem with corridors is the installation of a window at the far end of the corridor wall which can create extreme glare problems.

Create unobtrusive opportunities for social interaction

The stereotype of so-called social interaction in a nursing home is the dayroom with chairs arranged round a television playing to an uninterested audience. Social interaction should be encouraged but it also requires a degree of spontaneity and function. The programme should be able to recreate activities around which socialization can take place. Outside an institutional setting, social interaction usually takes place in a bar or restaurant, or consists of watching, as in the theatre, or spectator sports. Consider the options in a design for creating social spaces that can take on the images and functions of those everyday facilities that are lost within the confines of a nursing home.

Maintain an individual's right to privacy, choice and control

One of the key distinguishing features which differentiate a person's home from an institution is the sense that one has control over what one does within it. Dr M. Powell Lawton, an eminent gerontologist from Philadelphia, has stated that the degree to which one can relate and identify with one's environment and particularly personal space is connected to the degree of control one has over it. This implies the promotion of private spaces and not shared spaces particularly where people sleep. Semi-private rooms and special care units are not conducive to the goals of privacy, dignity and independence. Elsewhere in the facility social spaces should have nooks and alcoves for one or a few people to sit quietly and comfortably. Large so-called multispaces may serve large gatherings but where can one go and sit in silence to watch a garden fountain or a sunset without the feeling that everyone has to be doing the same thing within a group setting?

Emphasize links with the past and the familiar with a home-like setting

The move from home to a nursing home can be traumatic. Indeed it can be a cause of confusion and disorientation as a normal behavioural response. It is therefore very important that the environment reflects as far as possible images, scale, sounds, sights and smells of home to reinforce and trigger emotions and memories with the past. The images that will mean most to any resident may not be the immediate past but further back, perhaps to their childhood or teenage years. They are the treasured memories of their past life with those they have loved and lost.

Provide opportunities that support a programme for wandering

Wandering is not the same as running away, which is the wish to escape; wandering is a programmatic issue first, and a desire issue second. It is not sufficient simply to place a path for wandering within the facility and expect residents to use it. Also, once one has cleared up medication issues, there appears to be a residue of about 11 to 12 per cent of residents who can be described as wanderers. Research has identified three types of wandering behaviour

- wandering as a consequence of disorientation caused by a confusing building layout or the lack of any way-finding clues;
- learned behaviour, e.g. perhaps a habitual experience gained from a previous inappropriate environment;
- restless seeking activity where the environment provides little stimulation to satisfy or engage a resident.

Within these categories are further types such as roamers who may rummage through other people's drawers etc. In order to overcome the above wandering paths should pass through areas of activity and variety, not just into a courtyard. We must consider that while we often use the word wandering in relation to people with dementia, in a way we all do it – we all enjoy going for a stroll and observing activities, therefore why not use similar imagery in a future design. We might instead call it the need to take a stroll to walk the dog. It is, after all, a normal pattern of human behaviour to recreate the variety of a walk round the block, e.g. to pick up a newspaper, to watch the children playing in the park, to meet the neighbours.

Define spaces into public, shared, semi-private, private, staff, indoors and outdoors

Within any dementia care facility, it is possible to define and categorise the various groups of spaces ranging from public to private. Everyone should have their own territory which needs to be recognized and respected. The relationships between the groups of rooms themselves are as important as those between rooms in each group.

Spaces can be divided broadly into 6 groups:

Private: where residents live, sleep and dress. This is their exclusive territory with access restricted to the owner of a room and invited guests or staff.
- residents' rooms (if single occupancy)
- residents' *en suite* shower/toilet

Semi-private spaces: where residents may have to share spaces where they live and sleep or bathe or wash. Access is restricted to the agreed sharers of spaces, invited guests and staff.
- shared residents' rooms
- shared residents' *en suite* shower/toilet

Shared spaces: these are shared among members of a household or family group within a cluster arrangement. Access is restricted to members of the family group, invited guests and staff.
- lounge, dining and kitchen areas
- circulation areas
- assisted bathrooms
- shower and toilet facilities that are not *en suite* to residents' rooms
- any other activity within a cluster
- outdoor spaces

Public spaces: used by anyone within the facility. Access is restricted to residents and staff of the facility apart perhaps from day visitors and guests.
- entrance lobby
- central dining area
- lounge area
- outdoor spaces

Staff space: where staff work and rest. Access is restricted to staff only.
- main kitchen

- reception
- office administration
- staff rest areas

Utility: where things are stored or cleaned. Access is restricted to staff only.
- sluice
- stores
- linen store
- plant room

The interrelationships are shown diagrammatically in Figure 12.1.

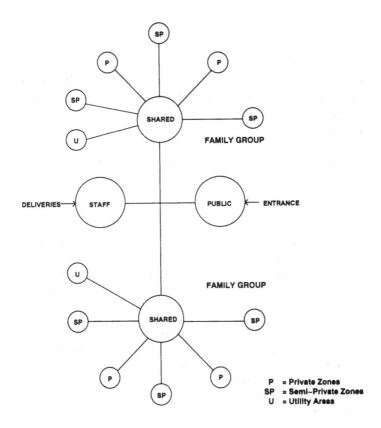

Fig. 12.1   Diagram of relationships of groups of spaces in dementia care units.

Allow for future change and changing needs

Organizational demands for both staff and residents are constantly changing and evolving, so it is important to ensure that what we plan for today will not be redundant tomorrow. Because the condition of dementia can vary from patient to patient, and vary in each patient over time, the key goal in any design solution must be flexibility. The building should therefore be capable of allowing improvisation and a change in which programmes are undertaken on a day-to-day basis.

As we gain a clearer understanding of how the physical environment can affect therapy programmes for people with dementia, so there remains a hope that the quality of life for even those afflicted with this terrible condition can be improved.

Conclusions

What is clear is that as a chronic condition, the warehousing of people with dementia in inappropriate environments based upon institutional medical models will aggravate the condition and squander staff time. Dementia is a psychological condition not a medical illness; its treatment therefore needs to be accommodated outside a nursing home, within a supportive and therapeutic residential environment. The care of this condition and the environments that will be required in the future for ever-growing numbers of dementia cases will present a key challenge to the financing of any health care delivery system.

References

Calkins, M. (1988) *Designing for Dementia: Planning Environments for the Elderly and Confused.* Owings Mills National Health Publishing.

Cohen, U., Weisman, G., Ray, K., *et al.* (1988) *Environments for People with Dementia: Design Guide.* Milwaukee Centre for Architecture and Urban Planning Research, University of Wisconsin, Milwaukee.

Cohen, U. and Weisman, G. (1991) *Holding onto Home, Designing Environments for People with Dementia.* John Hopkins University Press, Baltimore.

Dychtwald, K. and Fowler, J. (1990) *Age Wave.* Bantam Books, New York.

Hyatt, L. (1991) *Nursing Home Renovation: Design for Reform.* Butterworth Architecture, New York.

Valins, M. (1988) *Housing for Elderly People.* Butterworth Architecture, London and New York.

Further Reading

Lawton, M.P. (1985) An Introduction and Overview of Environment. *Pride Institute Journal of Long-term Home Health Care*, **4** (2): 1–11.

Chapter 13
The In-patient Hospice – Theory and Case Study

Martin S. Valins, R.M. Sovich and Gregory J. Scott

The concept of the 'in-patient' hospice programme is relatively new. The following narrative and description is based upon programming (briefing) discussions held between the Hospice of Lancaster County in the United States and architects Reese, Lower, Patrick and Scott Ltd in 1993 as part of the design process for the Essa Flory Hospice.

Definition

The hospice is a model of care designed to support the physical, psychosocial and spiritual needs of people at the end of life. Its goal is to allow the dying process to unfold with a minimum of discomfort, maintaining dignity and quality of life. Care is provided by family and friends at home or within a nursing home or special hospice care facility. Staff at the hospice, including nurses, social workers, chaplains and volunteers as well as physicians, seek to address the needs of family members in addition to those of the patient.

Hospice care is appropriate when traditional medical care, so often focused on cure and length of life, is no longer the best way to serve the patient's interests. This may be when medical therapies no longer offer a benefit to the patient, or when the benefits are outweighed by their accompanying burdens.

While cancer is the most common diagnosis among hospice patients, increasing numbers of persons with end-stage heart, lung, liver and renal diseases and AIDS, are receiving hospice care. Approximately 210 000 persons at the end of life, together with their families, are estimated to be served annually by some 2000 hospice programmes in the United States.

Hospice and other health care delivery systems

A hospice is therefore a programme of care and not a building. It is so unique in terms of the health care delivery system it offers that it does not always fit into what already exists in terms of hospitals and nursing homes. It can produce conflict where traditional healthcare programmes take place in the same building as hospice care.

Traditionally health care does not respond in the same way as hospice care. For example, if a patient has a symptom problem and is unable to manage it at home, the patient will tend to be hospitalized within a system which is primarily focused on diagnostic and life prolonging programmes. The hospice brings a new speciality of palliative care that has different methods of response. It takes a different mind set to allow a condition to take its own natural course. There is therefore an entirely different process within the chronic phase, i.e. within a nursing home, to the terminal phase in a hospice programme.

When a patient chooses to enter a hospice programme the patient elects a form of non-aggressive care and chooses to be kept comfortable within a natural process of decline. In palliative care one is treating the symptom instead of the disease. The disease is progressive and what one focuses upon is how to comfort both the patient and the family, as they cope with increased needs or imminent loss.

The traditional medical model deals with the patient and a medical/ physical problem. The patient comes to the medical provider on the medical provider's territory. However the hospice provides care to the patient wherever they are to meet their needs. The majority of care is carried out in the patient's own home and therefore the hospice offers care at the patient's invitation.

User profile example

A person may receive treatment for a serious condition which is treated aggressively. The treatment may do little to improve or combat the condition, and the disease is progressing. The physician may at this point suggest that this is a potential hospice referral. Although the patient remains conscious, there may be nothing further that can be done as a cure, with recovery no longer an option. Yet the patient may have symptoms, e.g. shortness of breath, and may require assistance. Here the hospice can provide support to the primary care giver. It goes into the home with registered nurses dealing with symptom management and perhaps arranging for a volunteer to come in and help with the shopping or running errands. The role of the social worker will be vital to work with the family during the transition from a curative to a terminal mode.

The setting for this hospice programme would be where that patient and family choose to be, primarily within their own home. However for the patient who may not have family members, or whose family members do not live locally, this can often put a strain on any informal care-giving network. In addition, some patients may suffer from difficult or unmanageable symptoms and unresolved pain. Family or friends may also require time for respite and need a place where their loved one can be cared for. The primary care giver may also be elderly, with medical problems of his or her own. The patient may be confined to bed, thus placing further burdens on the primary care giver. For these reasons the patient and family need to know which other options exist. The provision of an in-patient hospice centre can therefore be a resource and can add to the range of options to a patient's family and friends.

Theory (by R.M. Sovich)

Having worked upon the design for the Essa Flory Hospice Lancaster County as project architect with Reese Lower Patrick and Scott Sovich furthered his research by tracing the problematic temporary approaches to the design of environments for the terminally ill.

Specific examples cited present a view of current concerns and future trends in the design of in-patient hospices. A comprehensive shift in thinking for both users and design professionals is crucial for the development of patient-focused care centres. Clues to the future form of these environments may be found in the development of a phenomenological design approach.

The in-patient hospice concept in its present form is still evolving. As established in 1967 in England by Dame Cicely Saunders and later expanded into the United States in 1974, it has grown into a worldwide movement providing care for terminally ill people away from hospital. This fundamental premise runs counter to modern western thinking formed over the past two centuries, which views death as a failure and prefers the dying to be hidden from public view (Bauman, 1992).

Looking back

When we place the hospice movement in the context of other trends over the past 30 years a pattern emerges. The Americans With Disabilities Act (ADA), an extension of the Civil Rights movement and the Advance Directive laws operative in many states in the USA, can together be viewed as an attempt through legislation to transform our view on disabilities and people who have them. Under this legislation all public buildings in the USA must be made accessible and discrimination against a person specifically because of their disability is illegal. If the disabled person has specific rights what are the rights of the dying?

Birth and death

During the period since the inception of the hospice, the ecology movement which has developed in the United States and Europe revived collective concern for the natural environment and reminded us that humanity is indeed part of the whole earth.

Birth and death are a part of the natural cycle of life. In the words of Sandell Stoddard:

'having accepted the realities of birth as a natural process to be celebrated and respected we are now bound, I think, to have a clear look at the process of dying' (Stoddard, 1978).

This quiet revolution has also filtered through to the medical profession where childbirth procedures are becoming more informal and open to a mother's choice. Consequently the design of contemporary maternity wards is becoming increasingly influenced by natural and less medically-invasive procedures. Yet an appropriate change in thinking in the form of in-patient hospice care would be more difficult to effect because our attitudes toward dying are more deeply entrenched.

The modern view of dying

Although death is inevitable and natural, today we go about our daily lives oblivious to our own mortality (Rinpoche 1992). The dying are mostly kept from public view in hospitals and nursing homes. But this is a relatively recent phenomenon. 'In Medieval times dying persons were seen as prophetic persons, voyagers and pilgrims' (Stoddard, 1978). The medieval hospital was a place of respite for these weary travellers. Caring for the dying was a natural part of activities of daily life as caring for the elderly.

The modern rational view places humanity apart from, or above, other creatures on the planet and nature itself, displacing religious faiths or beliefs and dismissing as 'primitive' rituals which could not be expanded with reason. For a few centuries now death has stopped being the entry into another phase of being which it once was: 'death has been reduced to an exit, pure and simple, a moment of cessation, an end to all purpose and planning' (Bauman, 1992).

Modern medicine challenges the individual cause of death, if not death itself. Bauman (1992) has commented that to Western society

> 'death was an emphatic denial of everything that the brave new world of modernity stood for ... the moment it ceased to be tame death has become a guilty secret ... one does not address death any more as a phenomenon that is natural and necessary. Death is a defeat, a business loss ... when death arrives it is considered as an accident, a sign of impotence or misdemeanour ...'

The irony is that, simply put, without death there would be no philosophy, no culture, no religion. The inevitability of dying is the root cause of the need to find meaning in life, meaning often found in transcendence of death. The tomb and the monument are powerful architectural typologies because they transcend the limits of a single lifetime.

Great enthusiasm exists for the design of monuments. For example thousands of architects, designers and laymen submitted designs for the Vietnam Veterans' Memorial in Washington DC and subsequently also for the Korean War Memorial. The Albert Memorial in London's Kensington Gardens was a proud testament of 19th century gothic architecture commissioned by Queen Victoria in memory of her dead husband. Yet this energy is devoted to the already dead rather than the design for those who are dying.

It may not be coincidental that an extremely small number of designs for terminally ill people are recognized by the architectural community for design quality and contribution to the art of architecture. These projects are generally not considered as desirable or held to the same standards as other more prestigious building types.

Meaning

We have discussed several tendencies and movements coinciding with the hospice movement or in some way reconsidering modern notions. The period since the first hospice has been a time of re-evaluation of modern architectural theory and international style marked by Robert

Venturi's book *Complexity and Contradiction in Architecture* (Venturi 1963). The architectural community has, in this period, seen an extraordinary receptiveness to theory and philosophy. Karsten Harries suggests that this implies that architecture is in a period of uncertainty (Harries 1994). Architects have searched for meaning through semiotics, religion, history and deconstructivism but these ostensibly continue the rationalist basis for modern architecture.

Botond Bognar identifies two prevailing design approaches employed today: each in his view fails to account for the human experience relative to architecture. The first is that: 'productivist rationalism ... limits architecture to the aspects of how buildings are constructed and how they work'. The second states that 'formalistic rationalism restricts architecture primarily to the aspects of how buildings appear visually' (Bognar, 1989).

The first approach, when paired with those modern attitudes towards dying people previously discussed, often leads to this type of thought process in the design of a hospice room:

- start with the number of beds;
- determine the number of beds per room (say 2);
- align beds side by side;
- the resultant room size and shape is a simple addition of standard bed dimensions and bed clearances as prescribed by codes and regulations;
- the rooms can then be arranged on two sides of the corridor for efficiency.

This solution is a variation of a typical hospital model. This approach is safer than raising questions about what will be going on in the patients' rooms, or what will be necessary for an empathy for the occupants. Furthermore there will be no challenges from financing groups as long as the room appears cost-effective. Yet above all the hospice environment should look like, act like, and feel like home.

Embarrassment

There is often a peculiar embarrassment felt by the living in the presence of dying people. The range of words available for use in this situation is relatively narrow. Our verbal ineptitude with regard to dying is paralleled by our architectural ineptitude and embarrassment when designing places for people who are dying.

An example of this is found in some hospices where visitors enter the vicinity through a carefully planned canopy or porte-cochere, yet patients are brought in via the service entrance. The deceased leave spectacularly ungraciously via the service centre which in some cases is near the refuse bins.

It has to be emphasized that the administration and care staff of all facilities are caring and dedicated and are generally years ahead of the design community in terms of understanding the issues. Yet they depend upon the design professions to provide the appropriate setting for a hospital environment. Problems occur not only due to professional inadequacies amongst the design profession but also because of a deep subconscious fear and embarrassment about death. These can only be resolved by greater understanding of the needs both of patient and carer within a hospice programme.

Silence

The architect Charles Moore once received a commission to design a house for a blind man. He was selected over several highly qualified architects for one reason. He was the only one to acknowledge his client's condition and discuss the implications of designing for a blind person. Architects must overcome the general reticence about dying in order to find truly appropriate meaningful design solutions.

Alan Lightman (1993) provides us with a clue to the state of mind necessary: 'suppose that time is not a quantity but a quality, time exists but it cannot be measured'. In a world where time is a quality, events are recorded by the colour of the sky, or the feeling of happiness or fear when a person comes into a room. The time between two events is long or short depending on the background of contrasting events, the intensity of illumination, the degree of light and shadow, the view of participants (Lightman 1993).

Lightman's description implies that the potential for meaning and poetry in architecture lies in experience but not abstraction. In a hospice we must not think of a door as a product selected from a catalogue, it is an edge, a place where a son pauses before entering a room to see his father for the last time.

There is a silence for which we should strive. It is the silence which Juhamni Pallasmaa says 'turns our attention to our own experience – I find myself listening to my own being' (Pallasmaa 1994).

The next millennium

Since 1963 (also coinciding with the rise of the hospice) Charles Norberg-Schulz has, in a series of theoretical books, thoughtfully outlined an approach exploring the psychic implications of architecture. 'After decades of abstract scientific theory it is urgent that we return to a qualitative phenomenological understanding of architecture. It does not help much to solve practical problems as long as this understanding is lacking' (Norberg Schulz 1979).

Case study (by Gregory J. Scott)

Reese Lower Patrick & Scott Architects Ltd were commissioned by Hospice of Lancaster County to plan and design their new building in Lancaster Pennsylvania in July 1993. The process of design was to listen and learn, and above all to become sensitized to the unique needs and requirements of a hospice and the people it serves. The design was truly a collaborative effort between architect and client. The process not only enlightened us about hospices but brought a new dimension to our understanding of spirituality, healing and our environment.

The design for the hospice proved to be an opportunity to explore a phenomenological design approach. In the design of each patient room (see Fig. 13.1) we attempted to create a room with a centre which would accommodate various activities in a number of configurations controlled by the occupant, including solitude, gathering or receiving guests, intimate discussions, dining, sleeping, napping, views of the outdoors, and access to a private terrace. Each room overlooks a private garden and views from the bed were carefully considered as well as how light enters the room. The rooms were orientated to provide direct sunlight when it was most pleasant but without harsh afternoon glare. Three dimensional computer models fine-tuned this to allow for all conditions throughout the year. The flexible room layout allows personalization; it is the domain of the patient. Although the patient rooms are arranged in a line, they are accessed by a series of rooms which open onto the main circulation area. This provides views out and daylight in to the internal spaces. It is in essence a corridorless building where the concept and interpretation of home has been an important element in the evolution of the design.

The building inflects at the entrance to receive and welcome and it forms a dense cluster of elements enclosing two courtyards on a former cornfield and pumpkin farm. In silhouette the long roof lines reach

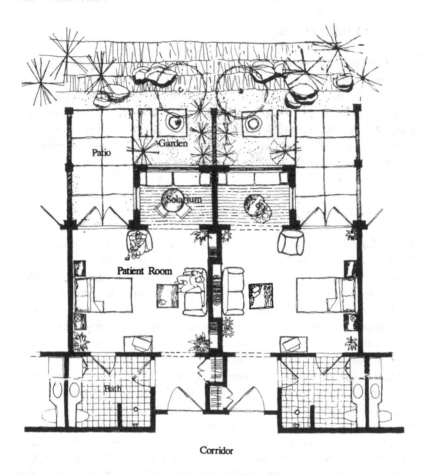

Fig. 13.1   Layout of patient room for the Essa Flory Hospice Lancaster County, Pennsylvania. A phenomenological design approach to a patient room. Architects: Reese, Lower Patrick & Scott Ltd.

towards the ground and although clearly new, it settles in comfortably with the agricultural conditions of the area. The building was completed in January 1996.

Conclusion

The hospice alternative has taken root throughout the world in just 25 years. It has taken that long to come to terms with the issues of organization, programme and identity. The next 25 years will find the identity of the hospice shaped by the quality of the facilities presently planned and under construction. Will the next 25 years produce thoughtfully designed patient-focused places supporting meaningful environments for more humane palliative therapies? The provision of good quality healthcare environments of course depends upon many factors, not the least of which is finance, but it is also related to our sensitivity to the needs of those who require care and their carers. The answer will depend upon whether those who finance and administer healthcare programmes, together with the design community, have the courage to listen and learn from the dedicated hospice movement and really look through the eyes of the patient.

References

Bauman, Z. (1992) *Mortality and Immortality and Other Life Strategies*. Stanford University Press, Stanford.

Bognar, B. (1989) A phenomenological approach to architecture and its teaching in the design studio. In Seamon D. and Mugeraurer, R. (eds.) *Dwelling Place and Environment*. Columbia University Press, New York.

Elias, N. (1985) *The Loneliness of Dying* (trans. E. Jephcott). Blackwell, Oxford.

Harries, K. (1994) Philosophy and architectural education from article by J. Pullasmaa, Six themes for the next millennium, *Architectural Review*, **1169**, July 1994.

Hospice Information Service (1994) *Hospice and Palliative Care: A Guide to the Development of the Hospice Movement*. St Christopher's Hospice, London.

Lightman, A. (1993) *Einstein's Dreams*. Bloomsbury Press, London.

Norberg-Schulz, C. (1979) *Genius Loci: Towards a Phenomenology of Architecture*. Rizzoli, New York.

Pullasmaa, J. (1994) Six themes for the next millennium. *Architectural Review*, **1169**, July 1994.

Rinpoche, S. (1992) *The Tibetan Book of the Living and Dying*. Harper, San Francisco.

Stoddard, S. (1978) *The Hospice Movement: A Better Way of Caring for the Dying*. Vintage Books, New York.

Venturi, R. (1963) *Complexity and Contradiction in Architecture*. Architectural Press, London.

Walkey, R. A lesson in continuity: The legacy of the builders' guild in northern Greece. In Seamon, D. (ed). *Dwelling, Seeing and Designing: Toward a Phenomenological Ecology*. State University of New York, Albany.

Chapter 14
Sub-acute Care

Laura Z. Hyatt

Introduction

Sub-acute care consists of health or medical services aimed at patients who may no longer require intensive care within a hospital setting but whose medical needs still require round the clock supervision. In the United Kingdom the term 'rehabilitation' is also synonymous with sub-acute programmes. Patients may be recovering from surgery or a medical episode such as a heart attack. Their requirements will therefore be a programme of rehabilitation and stabilization prior to a return to the general community.

The spotlight has turned upon this previously little known component of healthcare, due primarily to the offloading of hospital patients from expensive post-operative stays into less costly healthcare environments.

Sub-acute care was first brought to major attention in the United States in September 1993 by Hillary Rodham Clinton, the First Lady, in her address to the Senate Labour and Human Resources Committee as part of the preliminary hearings on healthcare reforms. Sub-acute care therefore can be seen as a healthcare format whose time has come, largely as a result of economic pressures, to contain hospital expenditure. There is nothing new or revolutionary in the concept of sub-acute programmes. It is just that the focus has changed and many financial observers are viewing it as the next big thing.

Patients who typically require sub-acute care are sufficiently stabilised to no longer require the services of a traditional acute care hospital but their condition is too complex for treatment in a conventional nursing or convalescent centre. Sub-acute care centres and programmes typically treat patients whose medical conditions require services that are intensive and technologically advanced. Less than 15 years ago the same patients remained in acute care units until they were able to return home or deemed chronically ill and discharged to a skilled nursing facility or convalescent home.

Sub-acute care programmes are currently provided in skilled nursing and rehabilitation centres in acute care hospitals usually in distinct parts and in specialised hospitals. In Europe the concept of the patient hotel described in Chapter 9 has developed sometimes on the same campus as a hospital. Within the less acute medical environment sub-acute programmes allow for and encourage family involvement. Therefore sub-acute centres can often be best located within the community affording greater access to family and friends.

The care available is comparable in many ways to care provided in hospitals with post intensive care facilities. Basic acute care capabilities are necessary for sub-acute programmes. These include a twenty four hour nursing staff with acute care experience, often with a specialization; a Medical Director: a multitude of ancillary services such as physical therapy, occupational therapy, speech therapy, social services, nutrition specialists, respiratory therapy and case management.

A wide range of services and treatments can be provided for patients with varied ages and diagnoses. Examples include physical rehabilitation, ventilator and pulmonary care, complex care, intravenous therapy, wound management, orthopaedic programmes, paediatrics, infectious disease, Alzheimer's disease: HIV related programmes, post-operative care and nutritional support. These programmes can involve patients with different complex conditions or focus on one area such as a centre specifically for patients with respiratory illnesses. This, that is, the component of ventilator care, is proving very popular in the United States.

Sub-acute care programmes are often housed in facilities that have other levels of care but are physically separated. In some respects these units resemble small hospitals. There are designated professional staff and depending on services offered there may be the capacity for ventilators, telemetry, piped-in oxygen and suction. Sub-acute patients often require both medical care and rehabilitation to achieve optimum levels of recovery. To meet these needs, on-site rehabilitation capabilities are available including a physiotherapy unit with technologically advanced equipment.

The length of stay in a sub-acute centre averages anywhere between 2 weeks and 6 months. Many medically complex patients face extended periods of recovery. Therefore quality of life issues such as the care environment are important. A less institutional physical environment is usually found in sub-acute centres. Design can contribute to a patient's ability to progress and increases the health care professionals' productivity. Fewer patients to a room, or larger room sizes, are necessary for the sub-acute patient. It would not be unusual for patients to use various types of medical equipment in their rooms for themselves.

The increasing demand for sub-acute care

Sub-acute care is increasingly gaining recognition as an important level of care, offering focused patient care and cost savings. It is emerging so rapidly that by the year 2000 there may be a greater need for sub-acute care programmes and/or other facilities than any other level of care. Purchasers, providers and professionals including those in development and design are charting a course for sub-acute care.

The demand for sub-acute services is the result of several factors

- rising health care costs have increased the pressure to regulate length of stays in hospitals;
- new technologies in medicine have resulted in the ability to save lives of patients who historically would not have survived catastrophic illness or injuries; and
- an increasing average lifespan along with new and chronic illnesses has resulted in a growing number of medically complex patients.

The rehabilitation sector of healthcare was the first to pioneer sub-acute care in the late 1970s and by mid-1980 other diagnoses were finding a need for a new level of care.

Standards and criteria of sub-acute care were being developed towards accreditation and many states in the United States had regulations governing its provisions in facilities. Sub-acute care was a billion dollar industry projected to generate over $5 billion in revenues by the year 2000. The same pattern of care is developing in the United Kingdom as NHS trusts look to providing more cost-effective programmes outside hospitals.

Sub-acute care is making a real difference not only in the quality of care to patients but also in controlling rising healthcare costs. These programmes provide care at significant cost savings compared with acute hospitalisation. Sub-acute care is typically 20–50 per cent less expensive than a similar acute care setting. The ability to transfer patients to a lower cost setting could achieve savings in respect of over 30 per cent of patients who are hospitalized. This saving is possible because sub-acute centres do not have the same overhead costs as facilities with expensive ancillary services such as emergency rooms, operating theatres, or trauma centres. By creating efficiency in the delivery process and providing specialized care, sub-acute centres are therefore able to provide quality care with fewer costs.

For purchasers and providers sub-acute care has become important as a positive method of managing care along with the associated costs of medically complex patients. Managed care providers were among the first to discover the value of sub-acute care. Purchasers and payers have integrated case management into their operations to coordinate both the patients' benefits and care. Sub-acute programmes also offer case management services which act in concert with payers and the patient's family to set achievable goals to arrange for patient conferences, revise care plans as needed in relation to patients' progress, to update the payers frequently and to see that the patient is moved on to the appropriate level of care as the patient progresses. Healthcare reform initiatives and the increasing use of managed care plans will contribute significantly to the future growth in the sub-acute care industry.

Design for sub-acute services

Lighting and the use of soothing colours are important. Space for pictures and personal objects should be provided. Due to the length of stay a patient may require it is important for the designer to be sensitive to creating opportunities for socialization such as common areas for dining and relaxing. Areas where patients can be outdoors such as shown in Figure 14.1 and spaces where they might meet family and friends, assist in allowing for a change in scenery and have therapeutic value in providing varied surfaces on which they might practise manoeuvring a

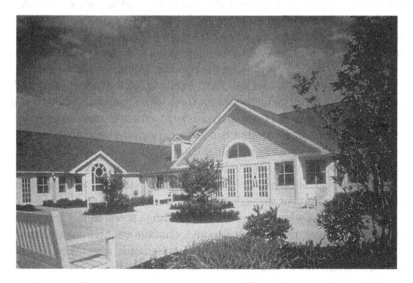

Fig. 14.1 Attractive courtyard setting can have therapeutic value. (Photo courtesy of C S & D Architects Inc. Baltimore.)

wheel chair or walking. Rehabilitation therapy rooms should be large enough to accommodate the necessary equipment in addition to whatever apparatus the patient may have to bring along such as intravenous pumps, walking frames, etc. Areas where there might be activity and noise should be located as far away as possible from the patients' rooms to allow for rest; this includes dining areas and kitchens.

A homelike environment that minimizes equipment intrusion is desirable. From a healthcare provider's perspective the nursing station and accessibility to the patient rooms is imperative, as are separate areas designed to meet the needs of consulting staff and physicians. Signs should be clear and directional. Just as there is never enough cupboard space in one's home, there similarly never seems to be enough storage space for staff equipment, the patients' belongings and all the extra medical paraphernalia that is needed in sub-acute centres because of the extended length of time the patient may need to stay in comparison with a hospital bed.

Sub-acute care in the future

As we look towards the 21st century many sub-acute care centres will be free standing as opposed to being housed in facilities with other levels of care or positioned on the campuses of existing hospitals. The physical part of these free standing structures will be like nothing we know today. They may even serve as a design model for other types of healthcare facility. Doorways to rooms where there are patients who do not require continuous observation will be erected in such a way that when open visitors cannot peer in, removing the zoo-like feeling that many patients complain about. The rooms will have sitting areas and couches or beds that fold into the walls. Families or partners could spend the night or stay for a period of time. This can allay anxiety and encourage an amicable setting so that a family member can learn care giving skills that can only be taught at night or early morning. Often after a patient has been discharged their healthcare needs become the responsibility of the family who may be fearful because of inexperience or lack of training in using the medical equipment that accompanies the patient home.

The sub-acute patient room will have storage space in the walls near the headboard of the bed that could contain ventilators and other respiratory equipment which is often cumbersome and takes up considerable quantities of space. This space will be easily accessible so that the equipment is readily available if required. As such equipment is often used at intervals or not at all, its storage has benefits beyond space saving, as it can be a constant reminder of illness to the patient when in view.

The furnishings and decoration of the room will be more homelike, for example with a table or floor lamps instead of intrusive fluorescent ceiling lighting. These facilities will also have areas where patients may prepare meals or do laundry. This will enhance the patient's functional independence as well as teach them to use assisted devices when performing daily living skills. Technology will have its role to play with staff and patients having access to high tech items throughout the facility.

Measurable outcomes will dictate that patients follow established treatment pathways. As medicine advances and the recovery process becomes more predictable, physicians will encourage out of facility excursions for patients. This might include attending a family function if feasible, or visiting other medical sites for testing. It is accepted that if a person is involved in routine activity a sense of normality is restored and progress advances more rapidly.

Patients will become more involved and knowledgeable about their care and recovery process. The desire to stay in one's community and to be close to family and friends dictates that these centres are located within that community. The needs of purchasers and payers and governments to contain costs, increasing sophistication of the consumer and advancing technologies available to the medical profession imply that sub-acute care will play an ever increasing role in the future care of the 21st century.

As the financing of healthcare becomes increasingly dependent on results, so sub-acute care is poised to become one of the most important elements of health care. It may also reawaken the opportunity for the skilled nursing facility as the long-term care market moves into assisted or close care.

It seems probable that as sub-acute programmes grow and develop and the nursing home population for long-term care declines, so the medical model upon which so many nursing homes were fashioned may become an important salvation. Thus the trend, which has already begun, for hospitals to form healthcare alliances with physicians, clinics and nursing homes will accelerate to form a more fully integrated network of healthcare provision with sub-acute care being a major player for the future.

Chapter 15
Acute Care

Richard D. Stuckey

Introduction

Nothing represents the 20th century's medical establishment as vividly as the modern acute care hospital unit. Over a dozen decades these have rapidly emerged from what Paul Starr (1982) characterizes as 'places of dreaded impurity and exiled human wreckage into awesome citadels of science and bureaucratic power'.

Imagining how such centres might look, feel and function in the 21st century occupies the minds of many of those who play a part in their creation. Yet with the next millennium fast approaching, realistic visions based upon a sound understanding of today's facilities and their historical place in society can lend an accuracy to future care. Such consideration enables today's planners and architects to influence the acute care environment of tomorrow.

Looking back

The earliest acute care environments of the western world were created during the 12th century by the Church in an attempt to prevent the spread of disease primarily through isolation and quarantine. The outcome was an environment that extended comfort to the sick and dying but offered little hope for intervention or cure. In confronting the overwhelming plagues that threatened whole communities the Church sponsored care, linking body and spirit. The union of church and state is reflected in Italy by the Florentine hospital *Hospitali Spedale degli Innocenti*. Built in 1419 it was a complex of cloisters, church and dormitories. Commissioned by a trade guild and run by the Church, it delivered a system of health, education and welfare for the community.

Health became recognized by the emerging governmental structure as beneficial to the whole of society. As the western world became industrialized through the 19th century, manmade environments contributed to large scale health problems, resulting in the emergence in the latter part of the century of a counter movement of hygiene, urging urban man to get back in touch with nature. In 1875 Dr Benjamin Richardson advocated a small hospital for every 5,000 people and the housing of mentally ill and aged in separate modestly sized buildings.

Throughout the 20th century there has been a succession of different influences on the healthcare system. During the 1940s the predominant issue was expansion to meet the needs of a booming population. The last 50 years in the United States have seen the implementation of the federally funded Hill-Burton programme of hospital construction. The United Kingdom's healthcare system was built with a similar infrastructure based upon a nationalized health service system. These highly regulated environments were designed for maximum efficiency for care givers more than for the human needs of patients. They are inpatient-based buildings with diagnostic, therapeutic and ancillary services beneath bed towers. A single monumental entrance typically leads to an information desk from which the patient is directed to registration, diagnostic departments, therapies and ultimately to beds. These diagnostic and therapeutic (D and T) bases became confusing mazes that forced some hospitals to paint directional lines on the floors to aid way finding. Once admitted to such a hospital patients found themselves in semi-private rooms arranged in a race track or cross pattern around a core containing support services and circulation. All this became a sequential scientific process which treated a patient as a product on an assembly line.

Civilization sought to control nature in an attempt to combat infectious disease. The acute care environment was required to juggle all of the financial elements and even control light, air and water. Public expectations demanded heroic medical interventions to overcome any affliction. The post-war spirit was fuelled by apparent victories over tuberculosis and polio and the promises of new technology. Heart disease and cancer were expected to follow. By the 1960s social concern for equal access to care identified the inequality of healthcare distribution. In the United States, while the Medicare and Medicaid Programmes addressed the needs of the elderly and the poor, this legislation also initiated the certificate of need (CON) process, the mechanism intended to control facilities and equipment expenditure in the health care industries. As an unintended ramification of CON regulations a franchising system emerged allowing certified hospitals to increase their market share, at the same time excluding competition and limiting distribution of resources. By the 1960s, 'for profit' hospitals in the United States outpaced the growth of even the computer industry.

Image and marketability came to the forefront of planning as hospitals competed for patients as informed consumers. While this was a trend set in train in the United States, it is relatively new in the United Kingdom with the formation of competing National Health Service Trusts. Building of too many facilities in urban areas contributed to healthcare costs which rose much faster than overall inflation. The need to curb growth is still with us.

Issues of today

Today medicine is too often practised defensively. Care givers are criticized over the overuse of available technology as protection from malpractice suits. Market conditions can dictate an aggressive response which does not allow time for the traditional programme and facilities planning process. Pressure to diagnose disease at early stages creates an ever increasing demand for state of the art facilities. Earlier diagnosis enables more care to be provided on an outpatient basis. The large number of inpatient beds built over the last decades are under-utilized. When the beds are justified, strict limits on length of stay are imposed. Individuals with long-term illnesses and no insurance have no access to a continuum of care when discharged from acute care. Yet inpatient beds at acute care centres and their staffing levels are too expensive for long-term care.

The redirection towards outpatient procedures and day hospitals suggests less need for inpatient beds. The beds that are required no longer need to be as proximate to surgeries and other diagnostic and treatment services. However new and acute diseases and the resurgence of drug resistant strains of tuberculosis are renewing pressures to isolate the long term chronically ill. Can the surplus beds in intensive centres be converted to sub-acute use? Not all existing centres have the space or flexibility to adapt. Again manmade environments tend to be less than ideal in terms of fresh air and daylight. While strict environmental controls are required for diagnostic and treatment spaces, they are generally too expensive and artificial to promote healing and housing and long-term application. Other shortcomings of traditional inpatient-based hospitals include proximity (or, more usually, otherwise) of services to parking and simple and direct way finding.

Have acute care environments fulfilled the potential of yesterday's vision? If the vision was a comprehensive healthcare system providing the best possible care to the whole society in gleaming white medical centres, they have not. Our high tech approach has passed many people out of the system. Today healthcare is too expensive for the market to sustain it. Acute care is, as in the past, more available to the rich and privately insured than the poor.

Planning did not predict today's huge volumes of outpatients and designers did not accommodate the divergent traffic types flowing to and between these services. Where inpatient centred complexes placed beds over diagnostic and treatment services, only horizontal expansion was available to house the growing outpatient services and new facilities. The resultant mazes were inefficient to operate and confusing and intimidating to use.

On the positive side, acute care environments have become active participants in the treatment of disease. They support technologies, research and procedures only dreamed of in the past. Excellent as environments to receive treatment, they do, however, fail to address cost effectiveness and the human and emotional needs of their patients.

Future programming and planning directions

Besides looking at the past, how can we formulate a vision of future acute care environments? Space requirements will be driven by the volume of service planning and demographic data. Responding to market pressures alone will not anticipate future trends or result in adequate flexibility. Future staffing needs and the industry's capacity to support the increased level of training must also be taken into consideration. This mirrors Dr Richardson's plea to revert back to 'high medical and human standards of medieval towns'.

Today we again need to restructure services around patients and communities. Patient accommodation should be provided as a hospitality service in a warm atmosphere. Acute care environments must be built appropriately. However, not all services currently housed in hospitals need to be constructed to the expensive levels of high tech services. Office buildings can adequately meet administrative needs and services like laundry, and warehousing functions can be accommodated in industrial buildings.

Medical campuses begin to make more sense than hospitals. Multiple buildings with individual entrances and identities can house distinct centres of service. Oncology, rehabilitation, obstetrics departments etc. can be largely self contained. Public wayfinding must be simple and direct in guiding people, often arriving initially by car, to appropriate

services. Parking with entry access will therefore be extremely important. Services will come to the consumer instead of being spread out all
over an intimidating building. The compact nature of such a design is
illustrated in Fig. 15.1.

Adjunct services will range from fitness centres to day care to long-
term care. Buildings will be tailored to their occupancy. Linking the
pieces together must be done in a simple and comprehensible manner.
Easy circulation is often the most effective way to achieve order so
segregating public, clinical and service traffic should be an essential
element of any master plan.

Future acute care centres will be planned resourcefully with emphasis
on efficiency, flexibility and environmental sensitivity. They will begin to
assume an active role in the healing process with expanded participation
in the treatment process. Artificial and natural elements will become
more integrated, with patients in control of their individual environments.

Future vision

What will our 21st century acute care environment look like? There will
be a polarizing effect to the acute care facility. Perhaps it is easier to
define what it will not be. Less primary care will be undertaken within
the hospital and it will instead occur more in lower cost primary health
care centres. Nor will the acute care hospital duplicate the resources of
academic tertiary institutions which offer highly specialized and
experimental procedures and diagnostics. This leads to a narrowing of
focus to simple and direct diagnostics and therapies aimed at the mid-
level of care. Strong diagnostic imaging, non-invasive special procedures
and general surgery requiring intensive care or extended recoveries will
be provided. Inpatient accommodation will be minimized. Taken to the
extreme this could result in motel-like accommodation with connective
clinical back up. Major resources will be focused on out-patient care and
series therapies such as chemotherapy, rehabilitation etc. If obstetric
services can offer quality birth experience with the security of clinical
back up, they will remain part of the acute setting.

We also see the acute care facility being the trauma centre for local
emergency medical services networks. Hopefully the public will have
options other than using emergency units for primary care. Depending
on the organizational structure of multi-hospital systems, the service and
support functions might all but disappear from the acute unit. For
example, in a more urbanized setting, one kitchen off-site may serve

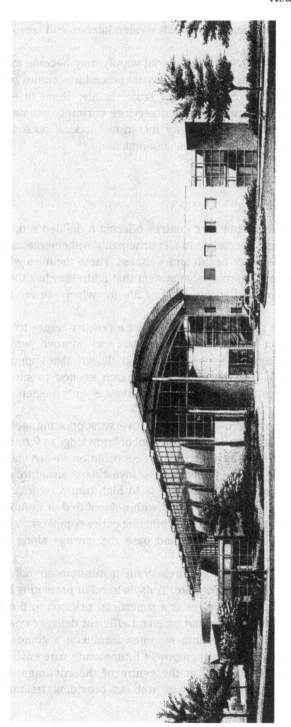

Fig. 15.1 View of new 'Fitness brings Wellness to Health Care' Campus. (OWP & P Architects Inc.)

several facilities leaving only a small scratch kitchen and serving points at acute care centres.

The 'just in time' system of material supply may become more centralized as the 'case cart' system for many procedures comes to rely on bought-in services if economies of scale dictate. Rural or suburban facilities will retain more parts and services currently encountered at acute care facilities, until density increases, making outsourcing or contract management of services economical.

Summary

Specially designed acute care centres offering a defined scope of services available and accessible to all participants will emerge as the new paradigm of interactive health and wellness. These facilities will be the central core of a comprehensive system that addresses healthcare as a continuum. After all it is the cycle of life for which we are trying to design.

We know that good design can project a positive image to the market place, attract healthcare professionals and improve performance and morale. Intuitively we recognize that design also supports therapeutic outcome. Yet the objective research needed to support our claims and empower healthcare executives is only beginning to be documented.

The healthcare system of the 1990s is diverse, supporting specialists in the field. Orchestrating the immense pool of knowledge to formulate and pursue a vision for the future is the best contribution we can make to the generation of acute care environments. Investing in structures capable of supporting expansion today will yield high future returns. Yet our current system cannot be burdened with unidentified or unfunded projects. It is imperative that we cease building entire complexes to the high tolerances of today's hospitals and pass the savings along to infrastructure investments.

As history has shown, large bureaucratic institutions are not the most humane way to deliver acute care. Today's trend of promoting hospitals as hotels and shopping centres is a superficial reaction to the age old challenge of reconciling human care and efficient delivery systems. To move into the next millennium we must formulate a grander vision. Sensitive planning today can empower future acute care environments to reach their full potential at the centre of the continuum of care, promoting health and healing as well as providing treatment and recovery.

Reference

Starr, P. (1982) *The Social Transformation of American Medicine.* Basic Books, New York.

Further Reading

Giedion, S. (1949) *Space Time and Architecture: the Growth of a Tradition.* Harvard University Press, Cambridge, Mass.

Mumford, L. (1961) *The City in History.* Harcourt Bruce Jovanovich, New York.

Ruga, W. (1993) *National Symposium on Healthcare Design Brochure.* Sixth Symposium, November 18–21, 1993, Chicago, Ill.

Chapter 16
Patient-Focused Design

David J. Kuffner

Introduction

This chapter is an architect's perspective on the evolution of patient-focused care. It addresses the importance of how a designer views the client and how that has affected facilities. Definitions and philosophies presented in this chapter are statements that are based on an architect's practical experience from study and work in the healthcare industry.

Looking back over the past 30 years – four examples

There have been four models of approach to the practice of patient care over the past 30 years as follows:

- team nursing
- the Frezen concept
- primary care
- patient focused.

There is a thread of evolution between these concepts that this chapter will explore.

Team nursing

The team nursing approach which developed in the early 1960s delineated the division of labour driven by experience and training levels. Team nursing was administration-focused practice for the health care system. Registered nurses were in charge of some clinical procedures, the administration of medicine and educational answers to any patient questions. A licensed practical nurse's role, though still clinical had more limited responsibility. The orderly's responsibility was a third tier of non-clinical general assistance and transport of patients.

The design of many nursing units took the form of a race track with the utility rooms, medication processing, cleaning and storage in the centre and patient rooms around the perimeter. The design maximized assignment of beds on a latitudinal or longitudinal basis given each team member's tasks.

These nursing units accommodated up to 60 beds due to the fact that most patients were admitted the night before a procedure and stayed for an extended recuperation period. The average length of stay for many diagnoses was as much as 10 days or more. Once admitted patients were expected to comply with hospital policies. There were strict restrictions on visiting and the patients were expected to stay in bed for quiet recuperation. Healthcare providers rationalized that such control of a patient would ensure a successful recuperation period.

The diagnosis and therapeutics services were consolidated into distinct departments, each having an independent need to grow. This independence fostered a reaction similar to that of a sibling rivalry. Competition for space, staff and resources was another symptom that affected the way that designers approached future expansion for each individual department. The potential growth of a department is illustrated by examples like the development of an emergency room to what is now the trauma centre. Patients were registered as inpatients cared for in the appropriate department and then returned to the patient room. This was a linear sequence formulating departmental layouts.

Frezen concept

Gordon Frezen was a visionary management engineer who developed a theory concerning the healthcare system during the late 1960s. The Frezen concept concentrated on time and motion surveys, material flow processes and the comprehensive overview of administered care. This healthcare paradigm is a clinical technician-focused concept. It elevates everyone's tasks to be viewed as part of the whole and as such worthy of the greatest efficiency possible.

In order to maximize the efficiency of highly trained people Frezen proposed that all the staff be geographically located according to their role within the system. A registered nurse (RN) was to be positioned near the patient's bedside for procedures, administration of medicine and to answer any of the patient's medical questions.

Frezen proposed to decentralize the charting system to the bedside and this in turn de-emphasized the physical nursing station and clerical functions by removing the clinical tasks. Placing the patient's chart at the bedside saved travel time to the nurse's station, thereby maximizing efficiency.

This approach even suggested that the food service crockery and clinical reprocessables be combined for washing and sterilization. Conveyor systems and cart lifts were employed to save time and increase the flow of materials through the whole system of care.

Primary care (nursing)

The primary care model was a reply to the division of labour seen in both the team nursing and the Frezen models. This philosophy retreated to the basics of total patient care. The primary care concept was a consumer-focused approach to the health system. The nursing ratios employed one registered nurse (RN) to six or eight acute level patients and one RN to three or four high level of care patients.

The primary nurse was reassigned to the traditional total care of the patient which meant that fewer allied support staff were required. The design implication was that pods, modules or clusters of patient rooms were more suited to this new approach.

Patient-focused care

Patient-focused care is the reaction of hospitals understanding the importance of becoming more competitive and providing a service that responds more to the needs of the individual and the community. The standard definition of patient-focused care is a design which places the patient in the centre of the operational policies. The purpose behind patient-focused care is to make the system simple and efficient for the whole patient which is mutually beneficial to both the institution and the community as a whole.

This practice is a way of rethinking the whole issue of skill versus task and makes a distinction in the responsibility of the nurse. Patient-focused care has a broader impact on the next level of an organization on a departmental basis. The concept of a department is being challenged from this standpoint and a department is no longer a physical operational entity that things or people pass through. Patient-focused care demands that services cater to the patient.

Case study

Rush-Copley Medical Centre, a replacement hospital in Aurora, Illinois has been designed according to patient-focused principles which embrace both staff and administration. The diagnostic and therapeutics departments have been arranged so as to separate the inpatients and outpatients, thereby simplifying traffic patterns. An outpatient can enter from the public space and have all procedures performed in a close facility while the inpatient enters via the clinical corridor. This facility was designed to break down the traditional barriers of surgery, cardiology and radiography to a high technology core of procedure rooms that have the flexibility to expand and grow over time. They share the levels of technology as the modules are tied together with an internal corridor. Figures 16.1 and 16.2 illustrate this.

The driving force of Rush-Copley is the fact that there is a sense of flexible order. This facility has been designed as a centre of excellence that focuses on the patient. For example, in the rehabilitation wing both the patients' accommodation and their daily activity spaces are combined but share facilities with physiotherapy. The departments have been placed so that their proximity will allow a patient to receive treatment without the discomfort of being transported several times. The Oncology Centre is another example of this efficiency of design. The linear accelerator is next to chemotherapy and internal imaging services are located adjacent to general X-ray of tumour growth monitoring. This does not duplicate costly radiographic equipment.

The Rush-Copley design has changed the format of the healthcare provider's role. Healthcare workers will be multi-skilled individuals, thus enabling a patient to check into their particular centre and to receive all of the necessary services, such as reception, registration, insurance verification and even billing, at the same location.

Patients' needs must be understood by the designer. Through focus groups and patient surveys patients often complain that a hospital is indeed a noisy inhospitable environment, where they lack privacy and are dealt with as a patient rather than a person. It is imperative to remember the patient when designing a healthcare environment. With this in mind at Rush-Copley, the entire site is divided into a pastoral, quiet side for patient overnight accommodation and an active side for entry, parking and access to services for the outpatients.

In designing an entire replacement hospital there will inevitably be risks involved. The first major risk at Rush-Copley is way finding. There are seven entrances to this hospital which makes it important to have a clear and welcoming signage and entrances that are distinctive enough

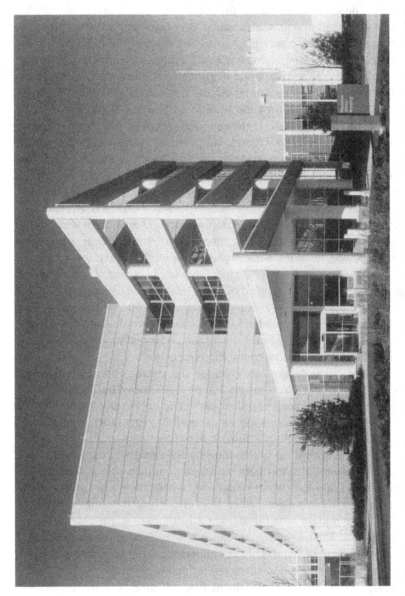

Fig. 16.1 Rush-Copley Medical Center: public entry to medical office building and hospital administration. The building has its own entrance and parking lot and is connected to the main hospital. Architects: OWP & P Architects Inc. Photograph courtesy of Howard N. Kaplan, HNK Architectural Photography Inc.

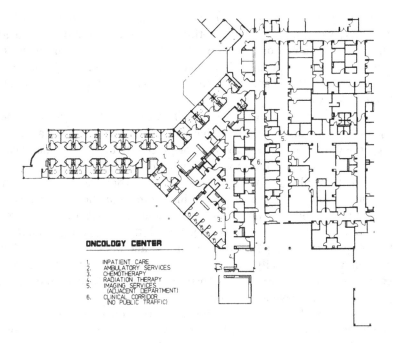

Fig. 16.2 Rush-Copley Oncology Center, showing both internal cancer care relationships as well as the adjacent imaging department.

to be remembered and described. Another risk is caused by the fact that this replacement facility is based on a new functional system and there is a danger that the employees of the existing facility might not embrace this new approach. If the employees do not utilize the system then the system will fail. If they reflect a negative attitude toward the operation, the public will accordingly form a negative impression of the hospital. We have seen many facilities designed and based upon one philosophy and being operated under another.

The future

We have come through a period of competition and expansion of services. Management is changing. As we approach a restructuring of the whole system of managed care, both in America and the rest of the world, in order to care for a larger population of people, we must strive to resist the danger of the system becoming an anti-patient focused model, because care providers will be expected to care for more patients with fewer resources. The revolution in healthcare will also mean that people's choice of care will not be as individual as it was in the past. The individual will not have the discretion of where they will be able to go, but patients will be obliged to go where their group has contracted for healthcare. There are models of care that work well in Canada and Scandinavia. We must analyse the advantages and disadvantages to learn from these systems.

We have come a long way to patient-focused care but we must set our sights on some areas where we have failed. We have not yet achieved control of inflation. There is inequitable access to care and primary care is not aimed first and foremost at prevention as a first priority.

Regulations always follow the test of time. Therefore designers and planners should not expect leadership from regulations. Regulations should be viewed as a minimum requirement, not goals to be achieved. We should not take regulation as a protocol. It is up to the clinician and the designer to develop new patterns of use and facilities which achieve efficiency and flexibility. Within that, the patient, the most important component of all, should be consulted at every stage of the design process via extensive focus groups.

In the future due to cost there will be a preference for the lower level acuity care to be dealt with by home care, recuperation and hospice care. There will be an increase in demand for the adaption of the home for a patient. With the highly acute cases remaining hospitalized, patient rooms will have better accommodation for visitors. This could assist the clinicians as the relatives will participate in care giving, thereby making them feel more helpful and involved. Cardiology, either treated with surgery or angioplasty will become more technology efficient and in turn will require a shorter stay. Oncology will provide chemotherapy and radiation on an outpatient basis. Tertiary facilities may become larger with intensive care, high technical diagnosis and a greater amount of experimentation and research. There will be an increase of secondary facilities to trauma care. General surgery patients will have a short recuperation up to three days in extended recovery centres. Primary care will be based on a 'store front' urban environment or a shopping mall-like suburban environment.

The baby boom population is now around 50 years old and due to the modification of lifestyles their life expectancy could increase by another 25 or 30 years. There is therefore likely to be an increase in retirement communities, inter-generational day care centres, sub-acute care facilities and in services to adapt households for an elderly resident.

There is the exciting potential for education and healthcare facilities to share space. This will allow students to get first hand experience and employers to continue their education easily. This would help institutions to cross train and keep skills up to date through continuing professional education. The negative connotation of a healthcare environment would be changed because of the energy and vitality which a school would bring. Community participation in health care environments could open up a new dialogue of understanding.

Healthcare is a service that is being run more and more like a business and so is being forced to jump on the information highway. All healthcare insurance and patient information will be logged onto a network database. In a few years patients will be given an identification card that will look like a credit card. This card will hold all the patient's medical information, for example when the patient received the last dosage of medicine. The patient's total medical history will be accessible by this card.

The efficacy of patient-focused care depends ultimately on its ability to attract public interest and confidence. Its merits as a system make it suitable both to drive the managed care regimes currently gaining credence in America and to improve the more rationed care apparently available in Europe at present. Patient-focused care is our threshold to a brighter healthcare future.

Chapter 17
The Healing Environment

Albert Bush-Brown

[This was one of the last papers that Albert Bush-Brown wrote before his untimely death. It is more conversational in style, but it reflects his rich and sensitive awareness of the difficult issues relating to providing a humane environment for healing. It was our wish that this chapter would be unaltered, and it is left as a grateful testament to a man whose contribution to the healthcare debate will be sadly missed. (MV/DS)]

The will to live

A spiritual reason to live is the most precious and delicate motivation the critically ill or ageing adult can sustain. But the will to live is not a simple motivation. In the film 'Shadowlands' the heroine cascades through fatalism, faith, love, humour, defiance, remorse and courage as she fights and finally succumbs to terminal cancer.

Most of us take the will to live for granted; we welcome each new day. But sickness of mind or body can erode it. Body and mind can devastate each other. Depression is one of the mind's mysterious devastations, so is suicide. But equally inexplicable is the jaunty joyful spirit we have seen in crippled and pain-racked bodies. What keeps the destitute, decaying, homeless person going? The mind, it seems, dances fantasies towards that peace which passeth all understanding.

Ageing can be a slow revelation of infirmities. Debilities and pain that decrease dexterity and mobility bring dependency which raises anxieties often inducing withdrawal and depression with consequent erosion of the will to live.

But many infirm and aged adults do not succumb. Instead more than just a will to live they have a will to grow. They want to learn to be useful, to enjoy and to give affection and love. What are the sources of their motivation and vitality? Just plain feistiness which kept one 88 year old invalid going after heart attacks and multiple cancers because he said he could not imagine a world without him? Or are vitality and motivation dividends of a genetic inheritance, the benefits of diet and exercise; or the legacy of a life free from disease. Do these bountiful treasures stem from kindness and friendships, from generosity and beauty, and even from spiritual grace?

The spiritual dimension

Today the sources of motivation in modern western people are far less likely to be the religious faith that prompted churches in medieval and Renaissance Europe to build hospitals, almshouses and life care communities. A sprightly 92 year old widower, the most popular dinner guest among younger couples in my village, when asked about the origin of his mirth and vitality, said he had been blessed all his life by wonderful women; first his mother, then his mistress and finally his wife. He said that he had lived by two precepts: always sleep with the right women and drink with the right men. The Church, he claimed, had played no active part in his life. Yet all of us who enjoy his company sense that a profound spirituality keeps him healthy.

Some preachers today claim to possess spiritual healing powers and no doubt their attention and touch may soothe occasional pain and anxiety but until one has repeated the miraculous raising of Lazarus or induced Francis of Assisi's stigmata, they will not inflict much of a dent in a market for CAT scanners, magnetic resonance images or chemotherapy.

Still, no one can ignore several millennia's testaments to the healing power of spiritual belief. Henri Bergson, a biologist philosopher, converting to Catholicism on his deathbed could not reason his way to believe in God but made a leap of faith and asserted that aesthetic experience, ceremony, ritual, poetry, music, dance and architecture were all springboards to that belief. The aesthetically-charged moment when all the arts support revelation is the elevation of the host in the Christian mass. That revelation moves some contemporary religious foundations to become exemplary organisers of healthcare communities. Their religious ceremonies draw worshippers to countenance a greater community and a greater power than themselves, sometimes through a belief in spiritual transcendence as a motivation to live through adversity. The bereaved also need reassurance, and familiar psalms and prayers recited within a chapel, as at the hospice at Boca Raton, Florida, provide that solace.

What if the spirit is not transcendent but immortality rests on man's good works, as for example Unitarians, Universalists and the Society of Friends believe? The latter have a desire to countenance a greater community themselves, and that there is a greater power than self- ishness is attested by the dozens of model life care communities the Quakers have established beginning with Foulkeways in Pennsylvania near the Gwynedd Meeting House.

The greatest legacy from the religious healthcare tradition is an ideal for nursing as personal care, indeed holistic care. That ideal was nearly lost to high labour costs and high-tech clinical medicine but is reap- pearing in the intensive care unit and co-operative care which enables family members to be in attendance. A model hospital for Saudi Arabia proposed by Spero Daltas allows families to live in courtyards adjacent to patients while separate corridors serve medical staff. An important contribution of the nursing cluster plan is bringing care close to the patients. Even in a dark and cluttered room the hand that holds has magic to comfort which no architect can rival.

The architectural dimension

One of the architect's fascinating conceits is that beauty inspires and motivates. Not only architects, but poets and painters too have attested that beauty has divine origins and the power to console, even to heal. We do not know whether the Greek father of medicine, Asklepius, believed that the golden section and his colonnade temple near the Acropolis were beneficial to health, nor Gothic builders their cathedrals. But we do know that the Italian Renaissance architects Alberti and Palladio ascri- bed divinity into a perfect sphere, hemisphere and circle and delivered a sense of harmony from contemplating churches generated from such neo-platonic forms. We also know that in the baroque age following Palladio, the circle was eschewed as a basis for planning churches in favour of the Keplerian ellipse which reinforced the Jesuitical insistence of communal worship at mass, not neo-platonic humanism.

Harmony with nature is the aim of meditation depicted in ancient Chinese paintings and the reward of pavilions and gardens in the Kat- sura Palace in Kyoto, Japan. To marvel at moonlight, to hear a ravine's awesome silence or to be lulled by a brook's ribbons is already to lose one's spirit from selfish bonds and to wonder about the origins and destinies which we cannot divine. Architecturally, harmony is achieved in manifold ways, but by way of example one has only to enter Le Corbusier's modern chapel at Ronchamps in France or a space designed by the Mexican Luis Barrigan, to sense a tranquillity that banishes anxiety and calms the soul. Their spaces are reverential, not clinical.

Where in the range of antiseptic interventionist hospitals and nursing homes, does humble harmony stand a chance? Healing through meditation is not in the genius of every architect, as meditation chapels at airports demonstrate. But Frank Lloyd Wright and Louis Kahn often achieved serenity in meditation spaces which healthcare institutions might well emulate.

The clinical model for healthcare architecture which is demonstrably successful for interventionist procedures does not salve the wounds of the large and growing populations of chronically ill, drug addicted, depressed, dying and dependent people. Spiritual harmony is a scarce or unknown commodity to many of them, and filtered light, noble proportions, peaceful sounds or a reverential space charged with mystery can help fill the void.

Reassurance, security, order and tranquillity are balm to the person traumatized by illness and loss. I once accompanied a long-term family employee to a well-deserved retirement at Meadowwood, a life care community. Widowed a year previously and undergoing chemotherapy and radiation treatment for cancer, with no relatives and unable to rely on errant indifferent children, she left her home of 36 years, sent her antiques to auction and entered a place that assured her of personal comfort and care. She was not at that stage interested in the social activities and artistic or intellectual opportunities which Meadowwood offers. She had had a premonition of mortality. She wanted the security of knowing that her residential expenses were contained, that food, laundry and housekeeping were provided and that her healthcare was insured. 'They even have an office for taking care of prescription medicines' she said. Meadowwood's atmosphere was calm, dignified, polite, orderly and serene. She asked me whether I thought she had made the right choice, and I assured her that she had.

The future

As the 21st century approaches, doctors, philosophers and legislators are troubled by ethical issues surrounding birth and death. Some issues like contraception, abortion and the termination of life have been in dispute for centuries. Other ethical dilemmas arise from genetic engineering, organ transplants and dexterity in prolonging life. Still others are moral issues, such as whether healthcare should be rationed to only some categories of infirmity or only to some age groups. Overall there is the question of who is responsible for providing universal healthcare.

Such questions will be bounced about among people who are immersed in a culture that combines materialism (the market place) with two motivations that are humanistic: perfection of self (physical, mental, emotional, spiritual, cultural) and dedication of self in service to society (work, community, charity). We are both selfish and altruistic. Our emotional life, including spiritual life, depends on that dual context, privacy and community, self and membership.

Deprive an ailing or ageing adult of opportunities to maintain this, as many healthcare institutions do, and the result is depression and morbidity. After surveying nursing homes for his mother one man called them warehouses for the undertaker. When deprivation pervades an entire institution, the climate of morbidity affects marketing and occupancy rates, personal quality and retention and ultimately financial success. Any life care community, nursing home or hospital so afflicted heads for a marketing expert, either accountant, management adviser or architect. However, it should first examine whether it has a humanistic embrace.

Are the ill and ageing occupants encouraged to learn, to be charitable, or to perfect skills or talents? Does it encourage them to be productive, socially active, and purposefully engaged? Or as in many, even affluent, nursing homes does the activities programme consist chiefly of abandoning patients each morning to watch television while their rooms are being cleaned? Are patients expected to be active, enthusiastic, aspiring, growing members of a vigorous community, even when restricted to a wheelchair, stretcher or bed? Or are they planned and programmed to be inactive, isolated, confined and clinically controlled – their day governed by tests performed and medications administered. Stimulating its patients to grow, both as individuals and as members of the community is also a healthcare institution's measure of success or failure.

Consider depression, a pervasive and recurring affliction. Its symptoms are well marked, among them: sadness, pessimism and anxiety, a sense of fatigue and disinterest, even boredom; distraction and indecision; hopelessness, helplessness and dysfunction; preoccupation with closure of life including death and suicide. Everyone recognizes some of those symptoms, because depression is a natural response to trauma and a transition after loss or failure. Helping depressed people make their lives meaningful is the purpose of Fountain House in Manhattan and nearly sixty institutions which are modelled on its programme of individual and group work projects.

Earlier, when I cited the buoyant spiritual grace of my 92 year old neighbour I did not mention that he is an art historian, nor that he is now nearly blind. Recently I asked him when he had developed his remarkable verve, which is more pronounced now than at any time during the 50 years that I have known him, even when his wife was living. 'When I was 82,' he said, 'I tried to understand Picasso; his images are awesome, I saw he was bigger than I was, he knew the terrible beast in us and the nobility also. I keep trying to understand. He gave me something to chin on.' Enquiry, wonder and growth provide a humanist basis for motivation which includes spiritual growth. Any healthcare or life care community that does not organize itself to promote its patients' growth as individuals and as members of a community stultifies and truncates them and advances them to senility.

In many nursing homes and hospitals the list of services and activities is minimal, encompassing little more than laundry, eating, meditation, cleansing and exercise. In life care communities that list is expanded to include entertainment, lectures, films and music and personal services, such as hairdressing and sometimes banking. The social ideal is passive, polite, seated, legs crossed, listening, but how can this provide opportunities for growth, learning and creativity? In contrast the humanist activities programme is based on purposeful engagement. Central to that engagement is the creative act. Writing offers many avenues of expression, particularly reminiscence. Painting and sculpture can reveal latent serious talent. But most arts and crafts rooms are inadequate jokes. The creative act requires studies and workshops so rugged that an anvil can ring there. At Medford Leas Continuing Care Retirement Community in New Jersey, one 75 year old in a painting studio enthused: 'I have never been so active in my life, I am still looking for a place to retire'.

Achieving the dream

What are the spiritual and emotional needs of a healthcare community? The answer lies in providing each member with two conditions: privacy and membership. Regrettably inordinate attention is given to privacy and much less to membership. That preoccupation is understandable. The private or semi-private room or apartment must be marketable and generate the revenues which the financiers require. Today in fact the private space is admirably planned, it supports the varied needs of its occupant, and surveys repeatedly show that this is desirable. We know how to make walls that separate people well.

What is less understood is how to make spaces that support membership. Many is a political animal and, perhaps Aristotle would also add, a social being. We cherish our privacies but also relish our membership. Membership first requires a community. A community is not merely an aggregation of residences. It has a larger scale of assembly and a shared social purpose. It requires gathering and work spaces and integrated connections among those public or common spaces. Therein lie the failures in most healthcare spaces. The public or common spaces are sparse, barely conceived and poorly organized. They support neither growth nor membership because they are not conceived to be a set of invitations to learning and they are not organized to foster communities.

Both faults reflect a failure to understand motivation; whether it is spiritual, emotional, social, intellectual or financial, motivation starts with purposeful engagement. Is it too much then to ask that every activity in each space in a healthcare institution be measured by what it contributes to purposeful engagement to a community that fosters diverse memberships and the motivations such engagements stimulate.

Measuring the motivational value of activities and their architecture requires fundamental questioning of each one. What for example is walking? Surely not merely taking a series of steps. Rather to walk is to roll up changing images, to pause and admire the view, to meet someone, to buy something, or to sign up to do something and to anticipate the destination. Each intersection may bring an encounter, maybe a conversation. Why therefore are corridors and bridges conceived only for striding from an inconsequential entry to a banal destination. Why not make them a social bridge that joins important events?

What is a library? What social functions can it perform? It is possible to get the mail there, to write letters, to listen to music, to receive a fax, to exhibit paintings, to take a message to relatives, to meet an author, to learn a language, to have coffee or tea there. Shall we congregate at a fireplace in the library before dinner, or is a library just for books, a random collection all catalogued and shelved behind a door which is locked at 5 o'clock?

When each activity, a bridge or a library in this instance, is broken out of its narrow confines and urged to contribute to a community offering opportunities for purposeful engagement, the old box-like rooms in healthcare buildings disappear. Why not make a social bridge of a congregational library as at Wells College in Aurora, New York. Similar social inventive thought is needed to free all the activity programmes from constrictive thinking. Dining can be a social and cultural experience. Gardens can be more than summertime enjoyment of bloom: they can be indoor gardens, clubs, planning spring planting beds at wheelchair height, scented gardens for the blind and gardens for all seasons where branch and berries cast shadows on snow.

A humanist programme relishes places for activity, studios to write, perform music, build cabinets, paint and sculpt and throw pots. One large high studio is best, though some creative work needs to be separated, like dark rooms for developing film and print. Too many separations readily lead to the boxing of boxes, each activity with its own locked door which destroys communities. Open the door marked 'sewing': the room is empty. But enter a studio and find a group clicking needles and chatting while painters and sculptors, each rapt in a personal intensity, ply their crafts.

What opportunities lie in productive work? Is the need to feel useful and respected for making a contribution to be curtailed when the ageing adult enters an institution? Or is there merit in enabling older adults to conduct day care centres, craft sales and benefits, to publish newspapers and to make gardens both indoors and out.

A productive and creative activities programme as described above summons uncommon architectural talent. Especially required is imagination with space and spatial sequence. As advocated by Bush-Brown and Davis (1991) special imagination does not end with proposing cubes, pyramids or hemispheres. Within spaces, refinement makes a space interrogative. A hierarchy of scale that joins part to whole, a redundancy of axis that creates spaciousness. How shall such spaces and their activities be organized? As now, too often a series of box-like rooms with locked doors on either side of the corridor? Or as concessions in pools of spaces along a concourse as in the Kendall CCRC in Longwood Pennsylvania where the passages open easily to wide activity areas.

Much debility and senility is circumstantial. They can be amended by a social and spatial environment that encourages both meaningful solitude and personal engagement as a member of a vital community. That is at least one source of spiritual reason to live. A humanist source with a life giving motivation, a reason to grow.

References

Bush-Brown, A. and Davis, D. (eds.) (1991) *Hospitable Design for Healthcare and Senior Communities.* Van Nostrand Reinhold, New York.

Gideon, S. (1949) *Space, Time and Architectures: the Growth of a Tradition.* The Harvard University Press, Cambridge.

Mumford, L. (1961) *The City in History.* Harcourt Brace Jovanovich, New York.

Ruga, Wayne, *National Symposium on Healthcare Design Brochure*, Sixth Symposium, November 18–21 1993. Chicago, Illinois.

Starr, P. (1982) *The Social Transformation of American Medicine* Basic Books, New York.

Chapter 18
Reusing Existing Buildings

Derek Salter

Introduction

What is an existing building? Is it that building which was originally constructed or is it that same building at a particular point in time? The question is akin to that posed by the carpenter, who when extolling the virtues of his trusty old hammer, stated that he had owned it for many years and in that time it had only needed two new heads and three new handles. Buildings tend to change from the day they are built, either by internal alteration and extension or even by demolition. The size of buildings may be restricted by site constraints, planning requirements or cost but the potential for change is limitless. We can extend buildings upwards, downwards or outwards to provide additional accommodation. We can convert by removing or relocating walls and floors. We can refurbish and renovate by making surface alterations and repairs, or we can rearrange by reassigning rooms. The point at which an old building becomes a new building is however debatable.

In Elizabeth Prescott's book *The English Medieval Hospital 1050–1640* (1992) it can be seen that the reuse of care buildings is not new. The English medieval hospital was a temporary refuge for the poor, sick or travellers and provided a spiritual haven for long-and short-term residents. It was not solely for the cure of ailments. Although the original basic plan was retained from the late 12th century, the open infirmary-hall arrangement was altered and as early as the mid 13th century some had private rooms. By the 15th century cubicles were converted into individual dwellings.

In 1610 James I granted a charter of refoundation to St Nicholas Hospital, Salisbury enabling it to embark upon a rebuilding programme. Some older buildings were demolished to make way for new rooms, a second storey with four rooms was added over the former north chapel and a kitchen was created for the hospital inmates. In 1635 the Chaplain's accommodation was improved by the creation of a new study and kitchen.

The next major step in the development of hospital buildings occurred two hundred years later. The Victorian hospital buildings pioneered by Florence Nightingale were innovative in their day, so much so, in fact, that 400 were built in Britain with as many others overseas. Many of these original hospitals are still part of Britain's present health buildings, having been extensively adapted over the decades.

With changed attitudes towards healthcare, rising costs and scientific advances, such buildings are at the end of their 'convertible' life, being too expensive to maintain or even to adapt further to meet current demands.

With the revisions to Britain's National Health Service over the past five years, it has been estimated that 20 to 25 per cent of the total stock of NHS buildings and land may be surplus to requirements. In 1989 alone over 100 hospitals in England were earmarked for total or partial closure.

The challenge of change

Many nursing home and residential care buildings in Britain are con-versions of Victorian and Edwardian buildings. Most of the smaller establishments were originally built as houses for the wealthy classes of the day and if their sites have permitted, they have been augmented over the years to provide additional residents' accommodation and service facilities. Historically, when hospitals and care buildings were originally constructed, no consideration was given to the needs of occupants in wheelchairs or those with mobility problems. The existence of floor level changes throughout many Victorian buildings, even by only two or three steps can cause major problems when converting them for care use. Frequently the original rooms are too large for single room use and too small to be subdivided. Because cost usually prohibits major alteration work the occupants are frequently forced to adapt to the building. In many cases the standard of accommodation in space and amenity terms is well below that which is desirable for the present day, let alone the future. However, much of the present day building stock in the UK, particularly of nursing homes, is of this type and without it there would currently be a serious underprovision of accommodation.

One question which must be asked therefore is whether older people will continue to accept substandard accommodation. The present very elderly generation have grown up less accustomed to contemporary housing standards and rapid technological changes than younger generations. Future generations of elderly people, however, will not be content with any such compromise. Those who have grown up in the 'consumer-awareness' age will expect all the lifestyle conveniences and electronic gadgetry to accompany them into old age. The standards of space, comfort and convenience which they have become used to throughout their lives will be essential in their choice of a building in which to spend their later years. Those buildings which cannot provide such facilities will gradually become obsolete unless they can adapt to suit the users' needs.

This process has already begun. For example over the past ten years there has been a change in attitude to the provision of increased privacy and private accommodation in residential and nursing care buildings for elderly people. Residents themselves and increasingly the children of residents who participate in the decision of where parents live, are also seeking higher accommodation standards in terms of dignity and accepted need.

For whom are we designing buildings and for how long?

Buildings designed to accommodate care provisions are used by a great diversity of people over the building's lifespan. It is the responsibility of the designer to provide facilities which will anticipate at least the next generation's needs, together with an element of flexibility for the presently unforeseen changes which will undoubtedly occur during the building's lifetime.

Clearly cost is a major factor in the procurement of buildings, both for new buildings and when adapting existing ones. Constant pressures are placed upon designers to reduce the cost of buildings. However, careful thought should be given to developing an efficient design which offers value for money, taking into account long-term staffing costs, future maintenance and energy costs and the anticipated life span of the building, even if this increases the initial capital cost.

Why reuse existing buildings?

In the mid 1980s The Economic Development Council for Building estimated that in the UK something approaching half of all construction output was accounted for by repair, maintenance and improvement. This stimulus for building reactivation has been brought about by various factors.

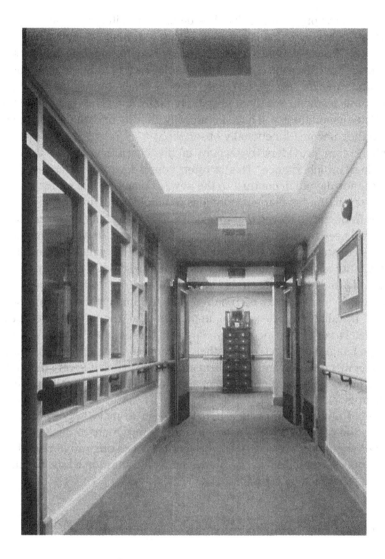

Fig. 18.1 Linkage of 'old' with 'new' in refurbishing a building.
(Architects: Salmon Speed, London. Photo: Crispin Boyle.)

A shortage of sites for new buildings, particularly in urban areas is a major factor in Britain, whilst sites in many rural areas are controlled by town planning policy under the so called 'Green Belt' legislation.

Planning and zoning controls also play their part in the preservation of existing buildings, such as the large Victorian psychiatric hospitals, many of which embody the best features of 19th century architecture.

They are now protected or listed as being of architectural and historic interest. Other uses for these buildings are difficult to find and they frequently cause disputes between their owners, such as the health authorities or trusts and conservationists. James and Noaks in their book *Hospital Architecture* (1994) state that 'It might be argued that the higher the aesthetic quality of hospital building, the greater the problem that later generations will have in radically altering or demolishing them when they become functionally obsolete.'

Many care providers, especially in the charitable sector, acquire buildings by inheritance. This is often coupled with a perceived preference for the old in contrast to the new, as many people prefer to live and work in the familiar surroundings of an older building.

It is frequently believed that to acquire an existing building means that little will need to be done to convert it to its new use. However, there are always constraints imposed by the existing structure which can result in inflexibility and compromise. Very old structures were not always built rationally and with modern day structural and fire codes major modification or renewal may be required. The full implications of new servicing installations are seldom appreciated at the outset and total renewal is very often necessary. Parts of the building fabric may be decayed and the effect of weather, dampness, rot, pests, structural movement, corrosion and vandalism must be arrested. It is very difficult, if not impossible, to renovate very old finishes to acceptable modern standards.

Should older buildings then be demolished to make way for a new generation of purpose designed ones more appropriate to the 21st century or should an alternative use be found for existing properties? The latter course should never be perceived as a failure or waste of time, indeed it is practical commonsense.

How does one begin to reuse an existing building?

The first task for the architect is fully to understand the way in which the users of the building wish to operate. This must include those who will occupy, visit, manage, staff, service, market and finance the building. Many clients themselves when instructing an architect have not considered these aspects fully and an architect skilled in the design of healthcare buildings will know to ask the correct questions to enable the clients to identify and clarify their requirements.

The main aim of the design brief should be to 'wrap' the building around the care services rather than force the users to adapt to the building. This is more difficult to achieve in an existing building than in a purpose designed building, given the multitude of constraints which the original building imposes at the outset. Nevertheless, it is no less essential.

Lorraine Hyatt in her book *Nursing Home Renovation – Designed for Reform* (1991) states:

'Participatory planning works. Effective design teams involve sponsors, staff members, residents and families in the planning process. Staff members in particular have important contributions to make to nursing home renovation.'

The future

When designing the next generation of care buildings, whether new built or upgraded, there must be more flexibility of thought both in the building and care programme design. We should be designing for every age group, with due consideration for mobility and approaches to care. Recent changes in the UK and the USA in attitudes towards access for disabled people into buildings has resulted in legislation which will

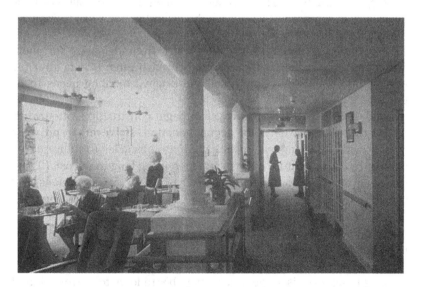

Fig. 18.2 Refurbishment of a nursing home for the Royal United Kingdom Beneficent Association (RUKBA). The area is broken down into 'family groups', with corridor walls removed to provide day areas and to reduce the visual length of corridors. (Architects: Salmon Speed, London. Photo: Crispin Boyle.)

affect the design of all our buildings in the future. Current indications are that this legislation will extend from public buildings to private housing developments as well as to existing buildings.

In many cases the changes necessary to enable buildings to be used by all age groups and abilities will not affect the able bodied. A light switch at the correct height for a wheelchair bound person for example, can still be used by anyone else, including a child and the elimination of trip hazards will improve safety for everyone. It should be remembered that with the cycle of life the young age, but the aged do not get younger. One survey finding in the report *Housing for Sale to the Elderly* (Baker and Parry, 1983) was that the most frequently stated reason for wanting to purchase purpose built retirement accommodation was anticipation of the problems that come with old age.

There is a need to reappraise buildings throughout their lifetime. Even buildings which were purpose designed for a specific use require updating over time. Healthcare buildings in particular need to adapt to changing attitudes of care and legislation requirements. Lessons learned from fires in buildings are passed on to prevent similar disasters elsewhere. Technological advances, especially in medical equipment, can have a dramatic effect on how a building is used and changes in market conditions and improvements in operational efficiency all affect a building's usefulness. There is also a need to carry out cosmetic upgrading to replace outdated furnishings and decorations to improve the quality of life for other users.

Very often the need to expand stems from demands for more accommodation, whereas the need to refurbish often occurs after the new additions illustrate how much the original building needs to be upgraded.

Building owners are always eager to begin construction, often when forced by an urgent need for accommodation. However, to do work quickly without a long-term plan can create obstacles to future development by barring future options and increasing long-term costs. There is a need therefore to understand the reasons for any alterations, and questions about immediate expansion should only be answered by reference to future needs.

An apposite conclusion to this chapter is provided by E Todd Wheeler in his book *Hospital Modernisation and Expansion* (1971)

'Everything that is done today may be redone tomorrow, but if properly done today, it can constitute a foundation, not an impediment, for the future growth which experience shows is inevitable.'

References

Baker, S. and Parry, M. (1983) *Housing for Sale to the Elderly.* The Housing Research Foundation, London.

Hyatt, L.G. (1991) *Nursing Home Renovation – Designed for Reform.* Butterworth, London.

James, P., and Noaks, A. (1994) *Hospital Architecture.* Longman, Harlow.

Prescott, E. (1992) *The English Medieval Hospital 1050–1640* Seaby, London.

Todd Wheeler, E. (1971) *Hospital Modernization and Expansion.* McGraw-Hill, New York.

Chapter 19
Towards a Conclusion

Martin S. Valins and Derek Salter

Good buildings don't just happen. They are planned to look good and perform well and come about when good architects and good clients join in thoughtful, co-operative effort. Programming the requirements of a proposed building is the architect's first task, often the most important.

(William Pena, 1987)

A new approach?

In order to plan effectively for futurecare we must adopt a new and radical approach to how we work in the process of healthcare planning. A goal must be to work within a more collaborative framework in which design professionals work closely with each other *and* with the user or client group for a particular facility. This will lead to healthcare environments which are better designed, take a greater account of capital and revenue costs considerations, and which are more flexible to changing needs over time. A collaborative approach will ensure that expenditure represents value for money both in the medium and long term.

A collaborative approach is a serious attempt to break down professional barriers in order to de-mystify the design process and to recreate a true team effort between those who design, market, administer, manage and use all healthcare environments. We simply cannot afford to keep repeating the same errors of the past. There is a universal responsibility to take a fresh look at how we go about designing future facilities and to take stock of what we have inherited. Each generation of healthcare buildings, whether newly built or upgraded, should ideally be able to stand upon the shoulders of past experience.

It is a question of tapping into the latent ability that is already there. There are often creative ideas that are rarely allowed to be expressed during the normal course of the project process. The collaborative approach can therefore help liberate the project team so that we can learn more from each other, become better skilled, and together be more creative.

In order to ensure that any errors in health facility planning are not merely repeated in future projects, we should look to how better to sensitize the designer to the complex but often subtle requirements of care environments. A holistic process of learning and communication between designer and user group might be further developed to utilize a largely untapped and rich resource of highly practical and relevant design information.

We are still in the early stages of interpreting research and bringing together the design profession, social scientist and user groups to communicate and become sensitized to each others concerns. There is a fundamental necessity for anybody embarking upon a project to spend real time unobtrusively watching how people use existing environments, as this can often give the designer invaluable clues which may not be available from any other source. The project team should be assembled with a group of say ten to fifteen users simply to discuss amongst themselves and with the design team, their view on what they feel works and what does not work.

Cultural diversity

Another factor which will also need to be addressed is the particular need and contribution of people from different groups and cultures. A working party set up by Age Concern and Help the Aged to look into housing for disadvantaged elderly people of different ethnic backgrounds in 1984 found that they suffered from the additional problem of not knowing how to obtain advice and help. There was also a lack of awareness among service providers, particularly with regard to housing needs.

The implication is that designers must ensure that any special requirements related to religious, dietary or cultural traditional practices are allowed to continue and flourish within the framework of the designed environment. There should be close cooperation with representatives from the various community groups concerned, as recommended by the Age Concern/Help the Aged working party.

In the United States many innovative care providers are recognizing that thousands of years of healing experience was lost during the European invasion begun in the 15th century. The indigenous peoples of North America had and have, a spiritual understanding of the link with nature and the healing process. This 'rediscovering' of ancient healing methods is a symbol of the rich contribution that all cultures can and should be allowed to make to our future care.

Long-term planning

Problems rarely occur overnight. Often, by the time a project team is assembled they have to deal with a problem that has been apparent for several months or even years, particularly in existing facilities. This, therefore, brings into focus the need for the project team to maintain an ongoing relationship with a facility. Regular evaluation programmes can test and define how well a facility is working in the light of the criteria from which it was originally designed.

Preventative architecture

Preventative medicine and the promotion of wellbeing can avoid the onset of serious illnesses and save both ourselves and the nation the huge expense of acute care. Similarly, preventative architecture creates opportunities not just for solving the problems which have been discovered, but more importantly to anticipate them so that solutions can be planned for and built into long-term budgets. It allows facilities to develop with a planned and coordinated program over time by trying to anticipate change rather than merely reacting to it. Long-range planning does not necessarily involve every solution being solved by a building. It could mean a revised management structure or a replacement or upgrading of equipment or materials. Architects, therefore, will need not only to upgrade and design new buildings, but also to understand how best these buildings can be used, and to be sensitive to resident and manager needs over time.

Space as a resource: value for money

When viewed in financial terms, space may indeed be identified as an expensive resource. The effective management of space will therefore need to become an increasingly important factor as new technologies lead to changing requirements for space. Energy costs may well rise ahead of inflation, and the politics of the care environment will become increasingly complex.

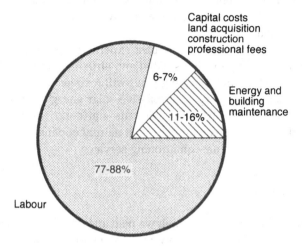

Fig. 19.1 Life-cycle costs of a building, projected over 40 years. (Original graphic by Reese Lower Patrick & Scott Architects Ltd.)

Getting value for money out of health and long-term care facilities in terms of space use has always been a puzzle and concern to sponsors and managers contemplating building new, or improving existing facilities. The rising costs of building, plus the revenue consequences of staff and materials will make it even more difficult to solve.

Just as a financial company will scrutinize its resources, so in the future, facility administrators and architects will need to cast a more critical eye over existing wasted circulation, uneven densities and space use.

Energy efficiency

Whilst it is generally acknowledged that at present, the cost of energy from fossil sources is not excessive and does not form a large proportion of the expense of most healthcare operators, it would be short-sighted to assume that the present level of pricing will prevail. The oil crisis in the 1970s showed how a disruption of supply can affect price dramatically and future changes in taxation on fuel and conservation legislation will always lead to uncertainty. Healthcare organisations have devoted much effort to reducing energy consumption for financial and social reasons. In future more is likely to be done to reduce dependence on energy both in terms of replacing old and inefficient plant and in upgrading or replacing buildings themselves. The pattern of energy use of large healthcare sites has encouraged the installation of combined heat and power plants where service heating is a byproduct of economical electrical generation.

New buildings, benefiting from past experience and rapidly developing technology, will be well insulated and airtight, lighting will become even more efficient and recycling plant will recover waste heat. Skilled building design will incorporate 'passive solar energy', with glazing to encourage natural daylight and with the sun contributing to heating needs, and there will be an emphasis on natural cooling devices to take the place of expensive air conditioning services.

Future strategy

If we look at the process by which we plan and design a project, we can get far closer to the core of how best to ensure that we plan for our future needs effectively.

Four key ingredients

- Develop a mission statement;
- be prepared to review the mission to remain sensitive to user demands and technological progress;
- understand the politics of development clearly; and
- view development as a cyclical and not a linear process.

These are ingredients that can help create health and care facilities which:

- are in tune with user needs and expectations
- are better designed to take a greater account of staff and revenue cost considerations
- achieve a greater capacity of adapting to future change
- take account of changing technological opportunities and medical developments.

Mission statement: this is the basic expression of why an organization exists, whom it serves and how it operates. A mission statement gives focus to the organisation. In time of indecision or conflict a provider should always look to its mission for guidance.

Without a mission statement there may not be appropriate criteria to choose between one option and another. The mission statement offers those criteria to enable choices.

Review the mission continuously to remain sensitive to current and future user demands and technological progress. Any of the following may have an important effect:

- demographics, age, income and health status
- medical developments
- technology
- overhead costs
- management systems
- future trends
- competition.

You may have a mission to serve a user or client that may be changing due to any of these.

Understand about the politics of development clearly: Reese (1994) identifies seven important factors:

- Identify the politics as to how decisions should be made – what is the chain of command?
- What are the sacred cows?
- Timeframe and budgets – set realistic targets
- Finance – how is funding to be arranged?
- Identify those issues that could stop a project
- Is the site available for development?
- What is the status of regulatory approvals?

Development is a Cyclical and not a Linear Process: When we review and evaluate how retirement and long-term care facilities are actually developed, we can see a cyclical process, illustrated in Figure 19.2.

The more one can appreciate that development should not be seen as a one off event, but part of a bigger picture over time, the better chance one will have to ensure that a vision for future care requirements will be achieved.

Seven steps in the cycle of development

Step 1 – evaluation

On first examination

- How well does a building or buildings accommodate/allow the mission to succeed?

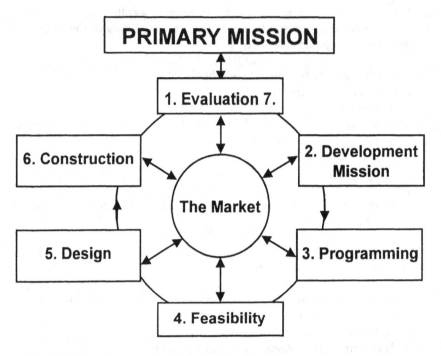

Fig. 19.2   Development viewed as a cyclical process.

- What are the inconsistencies between your mission statement and the current stock of buildings and services provided?
- Look at entire campus (not in isolation).

Examples of the above might result in the identification of problems, for instance, the mission may contain the desire to promote privacy and dignity for all users, yet a majority of your care beds are double occupancy rooms. Alternatively your mission may include the desire to tackle the care of dementia patients, but has no specific unit. The preliminary examination should also promote questions, such as how well are you serving users' evaluation surveys, or how well can the building support efficient and effective staffing/management systems?

The evaluation process can therefore provide you with the hard data to make strategic decisions. It can offer the opportunity for future generations to stand on the shoulders of past experience. Having looked inward toward yourselves, it is also important to look out – to study innovative models of care. Healthcare is in the midst of dramatic change, both in social and economic reform. It will be important to 'consider' the likely impact of change upon the proposed facility, not just from day one, but into the next century.

Step 2 – the development mission

The development mission statement is the basic expression of why a development is required – whom it will serve and how it will operate. It should, ideally

- list the issues
- prioritize the issues
- decide what can be afforded.

Capital costs tend to be viewed only as relating to the 'one-off' costs of development and construction in terms of square footage.

If one can create a more staff- and energy-efficient building design, the impact over the life cycle of the building will be far higher than if one only chose to focus upon one-off construction costs.

Step 3 – programming (time brief)

Programming is a process leading to an explicit statement of an architectural problem. It's the hand-off package. . . .

Programming is analysis . . . in analysis the parts of a design problem are separated and identified.

(William Pena, 1987)

The importance of project programming (briefing)

The programme (brief) should be an ongoing process which develops within a collaborative approach throughout the lifetime of a facility. The programme, therefore, cannot be viewed merely as one stage in the design process. Its interaction with both the designers and users of a facility should be continuous, rather than the more commonly observed 'conveyor-belt/factory assembly' approach to design for healthcare – that is, where the programme writer prepares a document which is simply passed to the architect who then 'interprets' the programme into a design. This in turn is passed on to the interior designer and then it is handed to the marketing team and so on. Last down the line are those who have to administer the completed facility, often without having been consulted during the design process.

A lot of time and money can be wasted in this way. A collaborative approach however, assumes an ongoing development of the programme, where all issues are evaluated in parallel and not in series. The architect should not be seen solely as the one who prepares 'pretty drawings'. Clients can become too close to a problem and thereby produce a programme in isolation which constrains the architect. An architect who is experienced in the design of care buildings can very often see alternative solutions to a problem if involved during the briefing process.

The degree to which a care facility succeeds can often be traced back to the quality and thoroughness of the development of the design programme within a collaborative approach.

The programme is therefore part of the conception and the very being of a project's design.

Design and function

In *Problem Seeking, An Architectural Programming Primer* William Pena (1987) notes that:

'The principles that apply to programming are to
(1) State the Problem
(2) Determine Needs
(3) Establish Goals
(4) Collect and Analyse Facts
(5) Explore and Test Concepts.'

Above all, programming is a process. The first meeting should be exploratory and expansive. At this preliminary stage take imaginative leaps outside the circle and brainstorm on a very conceptual level. Look as well at alternative plan form arrangements.

The result of the programming sessions should be compiled into a programming workbook which will describe

- What the healthcare facility seeks to do – philosophy of care.
- How it will function.
- Description of users.
- Description of each activity/space and its relationship to other spaces within the building.
- Computation of all rooms/areas to determine total estimated gross floor area – based upon the programme of requirements.

- Preliminary cost estimate based upon gross floor area calculations – as an early guide to construction costs.

Step 4 – further feasibility analysis

At this stage the project can proceed to commission

- marketing studies;
- site surveys; and
- confirm financing.

Step 5 – translating the programme into a design

Only at this stage should the development team begin to prepare design proposals and ensure that these are tested against the information we have – the programme.

The process of information exchange between the members of the team is maintained. Throughout the design process, the design is tested against the givens. These encompass

- the primary mission;
- the development mission;
- the programme;
- the design change;
- future change (user demands/technology/legislation).

Testing the designs against the unexpected

In the light of the above, one can develop some 'if–then' situations and test whether the design survives the journey. It is easier and much more cost effective to see if a design can survive a journey into the future rather than a building. If the design can 'fly' at the design stage – it will stand a better chance of surviving future change.

Step 6 – construction

The programming should be thorough enough to ensure that this phase can be completed as efficiently as possible with an absolute minimum of changes to the design. Therefore, while effective programming may extend the period leading up to construction, it can save time and money overall.

Step 7 – evaluation

As soon a construction is complete and the new facility comes into use, we should begin this cycle again, perhaps the most important stage in the process. Now is the time to ask how well does your building or buildings accommodate/allow your mission to succeed, and was your development mission statement achieved?

Futurecare

A definite trend to creating a healthcare environment that does not represent a technical approach to care, but instead embraces and supports the wellbeing of the patient/consumer is already under way. This, of course, follows a greater awareness of the impact of the environment upon the human spirit and psyche, in contrast to the technically-driven ideas of previous decades.

Our health is inextricably linked to the way we live our lives, and ultimately to how we protect and care for our planet. The problems of global warming through pollution and the breakdown of the Earth's protective barriers will affect the health and, ultimately the survival of all life forms for generations to come. Consciousness of the need to protect our planet is, however, beginning to develop worldwide in recognition of the need to preserve our natural resources for future generations.

This helps us to understand the recent shift towards a new philosophy of care in which the role of drugs and interventionist measures will diminish and the role of health care becomes part of a wider human experience. Many innovative facilities are now recognizing the benefits of using complementary therapies and drug-free environments.

Healthcare facilities can themselves be part of this new era in which buildings offering care are designed in the knowledge that we are linked not only to nature but also to the materials used to house us.

Healthcare and architecture are tending to place the role of technology in balance with more sensitivity to the needs of the human condition, the environment, and the Earth's finite resources.

The authors hope that Futurecare is part of the solution for a more balanced, integrated and holistic approach to the provision of future healthcare environments within the context of the finite resources of sponsors and in the long term the finite resources of our increasingly fragile planet.

References

Housing for Ethnic Elders (1984) The report of a working party set up by Age Concern England and Help the Aged Housing Trust, London.

Pena, W. with Parshall S. and Kelly K. (1987) *Problem Seeking – An Architectural Programming Primer.* AIA Press, Washington.

Further Reading

Getting Started (1994) *Planning For Care,* Report by Reese, Lower, Patrick & Scott Architects Ltd, Lancaster PA.

Additional Reading

Vision of the future relies upon thinking outside the circle and understanding and being sensitive to current trends and where they are leading. Yet there is no exact science to predicting the future; instead our own research has taught us that it is more a mind set than anything else. The following books offered a vision primarily based on intuition and understanding of the issues, and they continue to be a constant source of inspiration to the authors.

Toffler, A. (1970) *Future Shock* Bantam Books, New York.

Naisbitt, J. and Ash Aburdene, P. (1990) *Megatrends 2000: Ten New Directions for the Nineteen Nineties*. Avon Books, New York.

Dychwald K. (1990) *Age Wage: How the most important trend of our time will change your future.* Bantam Books, New York.

Califano, J.A. Jnr. (1986) *America's Health Care Revolution*. Touchstone, New York.

Directory of Contributors

Kenneth G. Bast

Job Title:	Consultant
Organization:	Hamilton/KSA
Profile:	Over 20 years experience as Vice President of operations in a community hospital, CEO of a growing trauma centre, Vice President of Health Services in America's largest continuing care retirement community and health care consultant with a national practice.
Address:	120 South Sixth St, Suite 1600
	Minneapolis MN 55402
	USA
	Tel: 612 378 1700
	Fax: 612 339 4477

Albert Bush-Brown

Albert Bush-Brown died in July 1994.

Chapter 7, The Healing Environment, was his last paper.

Albert Bush-Brown MFA, PhD, Hon AIA, was Chairman of the International Council for Caring Communities, a not-for profit foundation, (24 Central Park South, NY 10019. Tel 212/688-4321) which promotes integrative community planning. Dr Bush-Brown studied philosophy and art history at Princeton and Harvard. Before becoming President of Rhode Island School of Design and Chancellor of Long Island University, he taught architecture at the Massachusetts Institute of Technology. With Dianne Davis, MA, PD, he wrote *Hospitable Design for Healthcare and Senior Communities* (Van Nostrand Reinhold), a humanist advocacy of healthcare and design. Dr Bush-Brown and Professor Davis were writing *The CCRC, a Study in Communal Space* for publication by John Wiley and Sons.

Robert Dana Chellis, MPH
Job Title: Principal
Organization: Chellis Associates
Profile: Robert Chellis specializes in planning and financial feasibility
                   studies for lifecare and assisted living.
                   Publications include *Congregate Housing for Older People*
                   (1982) and *Life Care: A Long Term Solution?* (1990), Lexington
                   Books.
Address: 17 Windemere Lane
                   Wellesley MA 02181
                   USA
                   Tel: (617) 237-9436
                   Fax: (617) 237-1213

Laura Z. Hyatt
Job Title: Executive Director
Organization: American Subacute Care Association
Profile: Laura Hyatt has over 15 years of experience in the healthcare
                   industry. She was also part of the development team at Lifetime
                   Television. Dubbed a 'futurist' by international media, she is a
                   featured speaker at conferences on radio and television. In
                   addition to numerous articles, she is currently writing a book on
                   sub-acute care.
                   Tel and fax: (305) 864 0396

Joe J. Jordan, FAIA
Job title: Design Director for Institutions
Organization: Wallace Roberts & Todd
Profile: Mr Jordan specializes in creating buildings that provide for the
                   special needs of the elderly. His book *Senior Centre Design*
                   remains the definitive source for the planning and design of
                   senior facilities.
Address: Wallace Roberts & Todd
                   260 S. Broad Street
                   Philadelphia, PA.
                   USA
                   Tel: 215-732-5215
                   Fax: 215-732-2551

David J. Kuffner, AIA

Job Title: Senior Principal, Healthcare
Organization: O'Donnell, Wicklund, Pigozzi & Peterson, Architects, Inc.
Profile: David Kuffner, AIA, has focused his architectural career for 24 years on facilities for health care wellness. He has worked with over 75 institutions ranging from primary health centres, community hospitals to tertiary campuses. His role has included developing master facilities plans for both existing and new facilities as well as full architectural implementation.
Address: 570 Lake Cook Road
Deerfield
Illinois 60015
Tel: 708 940 9600
Fax: 708 940 9601

Amy E. Reese, MSW, RN, BSN

Job Title: Assistant Director
Organization: The Eaton Terrace Group
Profile: Amy Reese received her Masters Degree in Social Work at the University of Denver, focusing on gerontological issues. She currently serves as the Assistant Director at an assisted living facility near Denver Colorado. Amy also serves as a Consultant specialising in retirement housing.
Address: Eaton Terrace Group
333 South Eaton
Lakewood Colorado 80226
Tel: (303) 937 3000
Fax: (303) 937 3090

William M. Russell, MD

Job Title: Medical Director
Organization: St. Elizabeth Home
Profile: Dr Russell is a graduate of Georgetown University School of Medicine and completed a fellowship in internal medicine at Baltimore City Hospital. He is on the faculty of John Hopkins Medical Institution in Geriatric Medicine and has research interests in long term care of the frail elderly.
Address: St. Elizabeth Home
3220 Benson Avenue
Baltimore
Maryland 21227
USA
Tel: (410) 6443355

Derek Salter, Dip Arch (Oxford), RIBA

Job Title: Director
Organization: Care Design Group
Profile: Derek Salter is a Founding Director of Care Design Group, a
                 specialist health and care facility planning consultancy with
                 offices in London UK and Baltimore USA and he is also a
                 Director of the architectural and design company, Salmon Speed
                 Architects.
                 He is a graduate of the Oxford School of Architecture and a
                 Chartered Architect who has, for the past 16 years, specialised in
                 the design of health care facilities and housing for older people.
                 He is currently advising health and long-term care providers in
                 the public, private and charitable sectors and acting as director
                 in charge of building projects for the accommodation and
                 treatment of older people.
                 He has carried out extensive research into the housing solutions
                 offered by the United States and Europe, including Scandinavia,
                 and is currently working on several projects which will combine
                 this international experience to produce new forms of housing
                 facilities.
Address: Care Design Group
                 Tuscan Studios
                 14 Muswell Hill Road
                 Highgate
                 London N6 5UG
                 UK
                 Tel: 0181 444 1041
                 Fax: 0181 883 2226

Benyamin Schwarz, PhD

Job Title: Assistant Professor
Organization: Department of Environmental Design
                 University of Missouri-Columbia
Profile: Dr Schwarz has a PhD in Architecture from the University of
                 Michigan with an emphasis on Environmental Gerontology. He
                 designed several settings for the ageing population of the kibbutz
                 movement in Israel. His research addresses issues of
                 environmental attributes of dementia special care units, design
                 elements of assisted living facilities and long-term care settings
                 in the United States and abroad.
Address: 141 Stanley Hall
                 Columbia Missouri 65211
                 USA
                 Tel: (314) 882 4904
                 Fax: (314) 884 4807

Gregory J. Scott, AIA

Job Title:	Partner
Organization:	Reese Lower, Patrick & Scott Architects Ltd
Profile:	Gregory Scott's career spans 20 years and is focused on designing environments for the frail elderly that support their physiological and psychological needs in addition to the needs of their care givers.
Address:	1910 Harrington Drive
	Lancaster
	PA 17601
	USA
	Tel: 717 560 9501
	Fax: 727 560 2373

R.M. Sovich, AIA

Job Title:	Architect/Principal
Organization:	RM Sovich/Architecture
Profile:	Randolph Sovich is a registered architect involved in the design and planning of innovative facilities for health and care.
Address:	89 Dunkirk Road
	Baltimore
	MD 21212
	USA
	Tel: (410) 377 5487

Richard D. Stuckey, AIA

Job Title:	Associate
Organization:	O'Donnell Wicklund Pigozzi & Peterson Architects Inc (OWP & P)
Profile:	Richard Stuckey has nine years of experience working closely with hospital staff and administrators planning and designing healthcare facilities. Most recently he has been involved with the planning for the Rush-Copley Medical Center in Aurora, Illinois. This patient-focused replacement hospital opened in September 1995. Rick is a member of the American Institute of Architects and the Chicago Health Executive Forum.
Address:	570 Lake Cook Road
	Deerfield
	Illinois 60015
	Tel: 708 940, 9600
	Fax: 708 940 9601

Martin S. Valins, BA(Hons), DipArch, RIBA

Job Title: Director of Research
Organization: Reese Lower Patrick & Scott Architects Ltd
Profile: Martin Valins has considerable national and international
                 experience advising retirement and health care providers. He
                 has worked with providers in The United Kingdom, Denmark,
                 Sweden, the United States and Canada.
                 Martin continues to lecture on both sides of the Atlantic and is
                 author of numerous books and articles on retirement and health
                 care design.
Address: 1910 Harrington Drive
                 Lancaster PA 17601
                 USA
                 Tel: 717 560 9501
                 Fax: 717 560 2373

Margaret A. Wylde, PhD

Job Title: President
Organization: ProMatura Group/ITD
Profile: For over ten years Margaret Wylde has researched and written
                 about the changing abilities, needs and wants of an ageing
                 population and the criteria for effective universal design for
                 products and environments.
Address: 428 North Lamar
                 Oxford
                 MS 38655-3204
                 USA
                 Tel: 601 234 0158
                 Fax: 601 234 0288

Deirdre Wynne-Harley

Job Title: Consultant
Organization: D.W.H. Consultancies
Profile: Deirdre Wynne-Harley is a social gerontologist specializing in
                 residential and community care policy and practice. Formerly
                 Deputy Director of the Centre for Policy on Ageing, she is now
                 lecturer, writer and consultant/adviser to a wide range of
                 statutory and independent sector organizations.
Address: 3/15 St Germans Place
                 Blackheath
                 London SE3 0NN
                 UK
                 Tel. and Fax: 0181 853 2004

Index